MONOLOGUES OF A PEDIATRIC SURGEON

Dr. Alberto Peña

Monologues of a Pediatric Surgeon

Dr. Alberto Peña

Editor, James P. Cunningham III

Library of Congress Control Number: 2011905586

ISBN-10: 0-9846432-0-6

ISBN-13: 978-0-9846432-0-2

Printed in the United States of America

Book Design by Rebecca Sylvester

First Edition: June 2011

CONTENTS

DEDICATION

To all children born with congenital malformations and their loving parents.

To the new generation of pediatric surgeons.

To my children: Gustavo (deceased), Horacio, Ricardo, Tzatzil, Alberto, Alberto-Giovanni, Mariana, Emil, and specially to Dr. Victor Peña who has showed his unique sensitivity and expressed his desire to embrace this profession since he was 4 years old.

To my beloved wife, Andrea Bischoff, for her contributions to this book, her support, inspiration and generous love.

ACKNOWLEDGEMENTS

Dr. Richard Azizkhan

Dr. Andrea Bischoff

Mr. John Cardone

Mr. James Cunningham

Dr. Victor Garcia

Ms. Jennifer Hall

Ms. Keisha Isome

Mr. Dennis Kotch

Dr. Marc Levitt

Mr. Craig Ponzio

Mr. Michael Rose

Ms. Rebecca Sylvester

Dr. Daniel Von Allmen

Mr. Marc Williebeek-LeMair

EDITOR'S NOTE

Monologues of a Pediatric Surgeon is unique in its intended audience. Doctors, surgeons, and other medical professionals, no doubt, will be interested in Dr. Peña's writing but so will the many patients and families touched by his years of work and influence in pediatric surgery. Hopefully, those not familiar with Dr. Peña will also be inclined to read his story because it applies to all walks and circumstances and is a reflection of modern human life. To enhance the texture of Dr. Peña's narrative we included footnotes to numerous medical terms within the text. Although many physicians and medical professionals may already have such a vocabulary, it is important to Dr. Peña to allow those that are interested, a deeper view and understanding of his journey.

There are many quotations laced throughout *Monologues of a Pediatric Surgeon*. Most have been cited and linked to their authors and their beginnings. Some are Dr. Peña's own words. There are, however, some quotations that cannot be traced to a finite/ definitive source. We have noted such cases.

PREFACE

This is not another surgeon touting his prowess in the operating room, or regaling over the countless dignitaries who sought his care. Rather, *Monologues of a Pediatric Surgeon* is an honest and profoundly illuminating account of a preeminent pediatric surgeon's perseverance and persistence in challenging dogma, navigating the staunch silos created by many a "blind believer," all while contributing to greater insight and rethinking of one of the most challenging pediatric surgical maladies—the spectrum of anorectal malformations.

Inside *Monologues* you will bear witness to a life lived as art: The general surgeon will lament that he did not pursue pediatric surgery as a profession. The medical student will be moved to switch from medicine to pediatric surgery. And the pediatric surgeon will come to appreciate how she too can move beyond the levels of expertise she thought possible.

For me, the core message of *Monologues* is to develop your life as an artist creates a work of art. Doing so, you can reach new and better possibilities. Your life and career can grow to the scope and quality of the greatest masterpiece. And with that perspective, you can transform yourself much as Alberto Peña has transformed the lives of countless children throughout the world.

Eloquently and evocatively, Alberto Peña outlines the creative process in action, showing us what love and desire for one's chosen career looks like, how to cultivate it, and how that inspires him, his team, and most importantly his patients and their families. We learn that it is the sheer joy in the hard work of being a pediatric surgeon that allows one to delve deeper and deeper into that well of creative genius inside all of us. This is arguably the second most important message of *Monologues*, for the aspiring pediatric surgeon and anyone else, for that matter, venturing to make a difference in this world. Whether appreciating the significance of imagination more than knowledge, or having a beginner's mind that enables you to progress beyond advocacy to inquiry, it is here that Peña suggests we learn how to learn, to "suffer a minute of embarrassment rather than a lifetime of ignorance."

Peña's depth of compassion, empathy, and heartfelt concern for the life-long well being of his patients leaps off the pages. He not only shares with us how becoming emotionally involved with patients and their parents can inexplicably serve as an elixir, but also his path of learning to integrate mind and heart in pursuit of surgical excellence.

Early in the book we learn of a very personal point of reference for why he pursued pediatric surgery as a profession and, perhaps, how Alberto strove to be one of the most caring and compassionate surgeons I have known.

This is no ordinary autobiography. It is that and much more, for it provides strength, insight, and a path for any aspiring surgeon that is eager to make seminal his or her contribution to the noble field of pediatric surgery. Alberto Peña provides a model for surgical noblesse that rests on persistence, bravery, and conscious reflection.

Monologues of a Pediatric Surgeon is a sourcebook of wisdom and nothing is more elusive—yet more needed—in this day and age.

Dr. Victor Garcia M.D., PhD
Professor of Surgery and Pediatrics
University of Cincinnati
Director of Trauma Services
Cincinnati Children's Hospital Medical Center
Winner National Jefferson Award

INTRODUCTION

Perhaps, at some point in life, most people have the temptation to write something and feel the pleasure of knowing that someone read what they wrote and was influenced by their ideas. This is usually a fantasy, of course, mainly because it is challenging to write something new and original. Events and ideas considered relevant or entertaining to the writer may be irrelevant and boring for many readers. Opinions and points of view are extremely subjective. They are the product of very personal surrounding circumstances, which, most likely, are different from the circumstances of the reader.

I learned all of this throughout my life and, therefore, have always hesitated about writing a non-technical book. Eventually, I decided to write, only to find that there is a big difference between a professional writer and a dilettante like me, particularly when trying to write in a language that is not my native one.

I was born in Mexico. I grew up there, attended medical school and trained in general surgery and medical pediatrics. Eventually, I went to Children's Hospital Boston (Children's Boston) to obtain further training in pediatric surgery for three years. After that, I returned to Mexico and was fortunate enough to be appointed chief of surgery at the Institución Mexicana de Asistencia a la Niñez for 13½ years. During my time there, this institution changed names on two separate occasions. Before my departure, and to this day, it is known as Instituto Nacional de Pediatria. Subsequently, I was recruited to be chief of pediatric surgery at Schneider Children's Hospital of Long Island Jewish Medical Center in New York, where I spent 20 years. For the last six years, I have worked at Cincinnati Children's Hospital, where the Colorectal Center for Children was created to care for children with colorectal and anorectal malformations—defects of colon, rectum, anus and urogenital tract.

During my life, I was fortunate enough to make a contribution in the field of pediatric surgery allowing me to receive invitations from all over the world. I traveled to many countries: rich, poor, capitalist, communist, democratic, kingdoms, countries ruled by dictators, countries with different religions, customs and cultures. I received many accolades, distinctions and awards from hospitals and medical schools, as well as national and international associations of pediatric surgeons. I also received gifts from grateful parents, all equally appreciated, including eggs, oranges, apples, cheese and bizarre objects, such as swords, bells, machetes, religious objects, amulets, trumpets, hats, liquor, wine, jewelry, pens, watches, paintings and even an eagle. Each one of these items brings memories of a sick child and a tormented mother—sometimes a happy ending, sometimes a sad one. In all of these lifetime experiences, I think there is enough about human nature and behavior, at a rather universal level, that could be interesting to anybody, not only to those in medicine and surgery.

Since I grew up in a developing country and worked under arduous circumstances, I can appreciate the enormous privileges afforded to me while practicing in the United States. My success at an international level, though, may represent a motivation for pediatric surgeons, as well as doctors from other specialties, born in developing countries. My message to all of them is: Yes, it is possible! Go after your dreams!

The fact that I have been very successful makes me an extremely positive and optimistic person, with an enthusiastic message to share with the new generations of pediatric surgeons. A positive, optimistic voice may be useful in a time of increasing litigation, commercialization and bureaucratization of medicine and surgery. In a way, I feel partially responsible for the difficult working environment that will be left for the new generation. But I believe, to confront future problems, new, young, fresh mentalities are needed to develop innovative and original solutions.

In this book, I share some of the most important episodes of my professional life. Some of them have a deep philosophical, humanistic meaning while others are humorous. One of the manifestations of the imminent human existential collapse is realized when people take themselves too seriously, more specifically, when they think that history will be divided into "before them" and "after them." A really serious thing in life is a sick child. I firmly believe that it is essential to always preserve a sense of humor—it is not possible to deal with children without one. Without a sense of humor, children do not accept adults. Without a sense of humor, adults cannot understand children.

Being a pediatric surgeon reveals a very special set of experiences: pain, suffering, death, love and happiness amongst them. When caring for children, these feelings may happen in a very short period of time, often within a couple of days. One of the main traits of the little patients is how quickly they go from being happy, healthy children, to becoming very ill and then, amazingly, how rapidly they recover.

Pediatric surgeons deal with families of varying economical levels, with different kinds of ideologies, religions, and political and sexual orientations. Yet, everyone—parents, relatives, grandparents and pediatric surgeons—joins together when geared by a common strong force: the determination to cure a suffering child.

Many years ago, I learned that most people do not like to hear advice. I also learned that senior individuals love to give advice, even when it is not welcome. With this being said, I hope that some of my experiences may be found useful, since one can always learn by observing another's pathway.

Finally, I want to share with my colleagues, mainly young pediatric surgeons and non-medical readers, my vision of the future in medicine. More than a prediction, it is simply my wish for what I would like it to be. I will feel very honored and privileged to learn that some readers laughed, some were moved, and yet others became excited after reading this book.

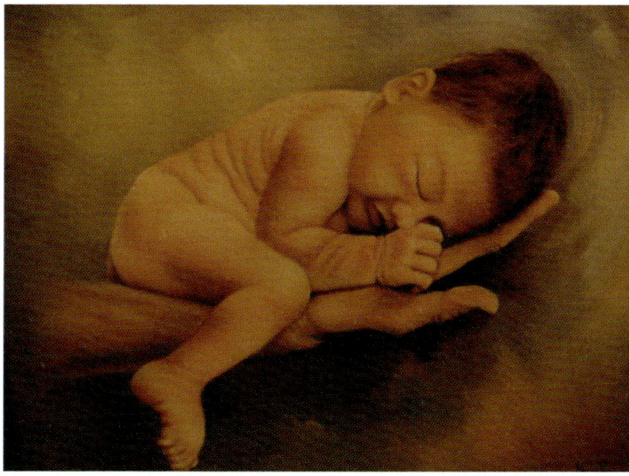

The Opportunity to Live by Mercedes Martinez

THE JOY OF BEING A PEDIATRIC SURGEON

Being a physician represents a privilege. Being able to alleviate suffering and make a difference in the quality of life of another human being represents an honor. The paradigm that motivates many people to become pediatric surgeons is the possibility to be a protagonist and crucial factor in saving sick children from lethal conditions or by improving their quality of life.

When a president of a country leaves office, for the following 20, 50 or 100 years, a controversy continues as to whether or not he was beneficial for the country. When a surgeon operates on a patient with a relatively simple problem, makes rounds the next day and sees the patient smiling, there is no dispute that they improved a human life. In sacred texts of some of the major religions, there is something written about the importance of saving a single life:

Saving one life is like saving all humanity.

It is frequently said that there are multiple sacrifices and restrictions imposed on a surgeon's life, including long working hours and limited time to enjoy their families, sports and hobbies. I disagree. I believe that the practice of medicine and surgery is a pleasure for those born with the vocation for this profession and, ideally, only those who believe this should be encouraged to continue. Humorously, I like to say:

Surgeons are divided into those who enjoy surgery and those who suffer practicing surgery.

I have not seen good, creative surgeons amongst the last group.

Select a job that you love, and you will
never have to work a day in your life.

—*Confucius*

*****

This is an era of extraordinarily fast communication. A multitude of events are rapidly relayed to people with impressive, spectacular images through the fantastic modern media. Many times these stories are presented in an alarmist way, provoking a kind of modern, neurotic state of mind. The public is accustomed to seeing wars broadcasted instantaneously. Many people witnessed, firsthand, the destruction of the Twin Towers in New York on that fatidic September 11th. Within minutes, the impact of an earthquake, tsunami or hurricane occurring in one part of the globe, is felt in another. At the very least, people are startled when they hear that the planet is warming, dwelling on future disastrous consequences of this seemingly non-stoppable phenomenon. They are concerned about the spread of a virus that is killing people in other countries or in their own. Everywhere, societies feel the consequences of the ups and downs of the economy and dread the potential collapse of their economic system.

Nevertheless, doctors must continue going to work in a hospital—a very special place where children and their parents endure—confronting serious diseases that are frequently incurable, departing a very poor future for the child. It is in the operating room (OR) or hospital ward where a very unique perspective of the world's problems is granted. It is in the hospital, while trying to cure a sick child, that the entire world and all its calamities seem to be less relevant. The center of the universe is that little space where a young human being is in pain and his parents contemplate him, invaded by all of the worst torments. The rest of the world seems to be rotating around the place where the child's life is at stake. It is there, where surgeons are humbled, recognizing that their personal worries and concerns are pedestrian and frivolous. It is there, next to a very sick child and his beleaguered parents, that the great honor and privilege of being a pediatric surgeon is understood. Most importantly, the possibility to do something effective with immediate positive results for another human being is there, within reach.

Any potential personal contribution to improve national economical problems, the contamination of the world, the heating of the planet, terrorism and other global crises, appears to be minimal. Doctors that excessively occupy themselves with formulating speculative solutions for complex, multi-factorial, national or universal problems, beyond their area of expertise, may distract themselves from their surgical work, preventing an emphasis on healing. Doctors must spend their energies thinking of what can be done to improve a patient and should trust, for instance, that economists are focusing on how to improve the economy. In theory, if all professionals in every profession concentrated on doing their best work everyday, the world would be a better place.

Daily adverse events in doctors' private lives may produce anguish and anxiety conspiring to make them unhappy. But again, facing true critical problems, such as a sick child and even more, a child who cannot be cured, helps to keep things in perspective. These events help doctors avoid becoming overwhelmed so they can give more realistic, less dramatic, relevance to everyday predicaments, differentiating the trivial from the essential.

At some point, doctors everywhere will occupy the patient's seat, because they are ill or because a family member has a serious medical problem. This demonstrates just how important the figure of a physician is. If that physician is also a surgeon, the scenario changes a bit. When someone allows another human being to surgically intrude and intervene in their body (or in that of a loved one), it requires a declaration of confidence, trust and faith. That person is elevated to an almost superhuman level. This encounter certainly influences doctors' lives. Doctors should always remember to behave as the person *they* would allow to open their body, to manipulate their internal organs and make life and death decisions while trying to repair their surgical condition.

All of this is true for physicians and surgeons; however, for pediatric surgeons, another dimension with its own unique features is introduced. First of all, pediatric patients represent a spectrum that goes from what is now known as "mini preemie"[1]

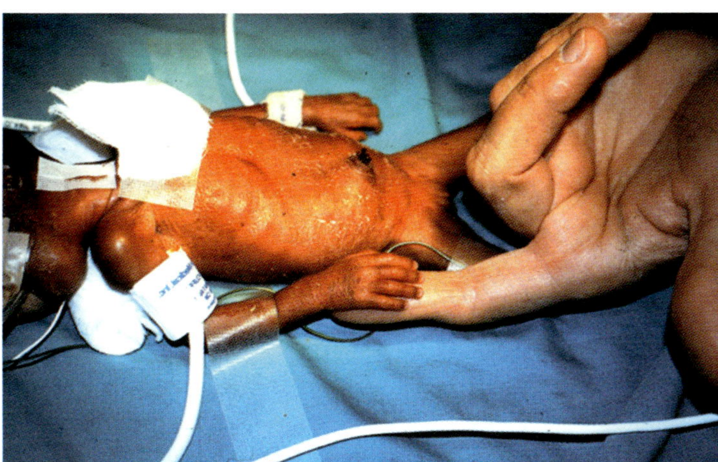

MIni preemie

to adolescents in the other extreme. In each one of these stages of growth and development, pediatric surgeons have to suspect,

1 Babies as small as 500 grams of body weight.

diagnose and treat conditions that occur more often during a particular age. A single symptom, such as abdominal pain, has a completely different meaning and diagnostic implication depending on the patient's age and gender. Examination of the abdomen in a premature baby with a potential surgical condition requires delicate maneuvers and a special awareness to perceive the baby's reaction. With a single finger, the surgeon should touch the abdomen and look for the manifestations of pain exhibited by the baby. A few minutes after that examination, the surgeon may be called to the emergency room (ER) to see an adolescent patient with serious abdominal trauma. The doctor's attitude and reflexes must change completely, ready to make quick decisions, under demanding circumstances in a rather noisy, erratic environment.

Pediatric surgery is the most curative of all medical and surgical specialties. There is no other medical profession in which a doctor is called to see a baby born with a lethal condition (when not treated) and within hours after a delicate operation, the little patient begins to have a normal life. Not acting adequately and timely, though, represents a risk of death or serious sequela[2] for life.

Adult medicine and surgery journals claim that a five-year survival rate, after a surgical procedure, is a success. In pediatric surgery there is about a 75-year survival rate! When a 70-year-old patient has a complication after an operation, she may have a problem for the next few years. In dealing with children, the

2 Any abnormal condition that follows and is the result of a disease, treatment or injury.

suffering may remain for life—a grim and constant reminder about surgical mistakes.

Operating on children offers doctors an advantage because they are manipulating otherwise healthy young tissue with an incredible capacity for regeneration and healing. Additionally, the majority of young patients are not obese, which makes operating easier and allows better results as compared with those obtained in similar operations performed in overweight adult patients. As a professor of mine used to say:

> *Children and babies are tough. Sometimes it seems like we almost try to kill them and yet they survive.*

A practical characteristic of this beautiful specialty is that it is one of the last real general surgical specialties. While adult general surgeons are becoming more and more specialized in specific anatomic areas, pediatric surgeons are frequently involved in all areas, including thoracic, cervical, abdominal, musculoskeletal and oncologic operations.

Besides their own well-being and family's happiness, what satisfies a doctor at the end of the day is to see that their patients recover successfully. Being a doctor, a surgeon, and even more, being a pediatric surgeon offers a unique position in society. This profession includes daily confrontation with life and death situations and the authority and responsibility of making decisions affecting the quality of life for a human being. Doctors are allowed to see the world and society from different angles, providing a more humane and wide perspective of the world's problems.

THE ULTIMATE MOTIVATION

The ultimate motivation for me to practice pediatric surgery, as humanistically as possible, was that my first son was born with an incurable congenital malformation.

When I was an intern in Mexico, I already knew that I would be working solely with children because I was convinced that I loved them. I decided to buy a book by Dr. Robert E. Gross entitled, *The Surgery of Infancy and Childhood* (Ref. 1) and I read it a few months before my first son was born. I specifically remember reading the chapter on a condition known as biliary atresia[2] and being very impressed learning about that terrible condition. Dr. Gross described that the disease was practically incurable. Newborn babies with jaundice[3] were studied in order to make differential diagnoses

2 Blockage in ducts that carry bile from the liver to the gallbladder and the intestine.

3 Staining of the skin and eyes by abnormally high levels of the bile pigment bilirubin (red bile pigment derived from the degradation of hemoglobin during the normal and abnormal destruction of red blood cells) in the blood.

between a hematologic condition,[4] a hepatocellular disease[5] or obstructive jaundice.[6] If the baby demonstrated having obstructive jaundice, he was all but doomed. Dr. Gross recommended surgically exploring the patient with hopes of discovering a form of obstruction that could be repaired. Dismally, less than 5% of these children were born with dilated bile ducts[7] that could be anastomosed[8] to the bowel, ultimately curing the baby.

Then my son was born. He was a beautiful child and we called him Gustavo. He was a little underweight and looked rather pale. About a month later, he developed jaundice. I first wishfully thought that he had what is called physiologic jaundice—a benign functional disorder in newborns caused by immaturity of the liver that lasts only for a few weeks. Every morning I woke up hoping to see that the yellow color of his skin was disappearing. Unfortunately, his jaundice was increasing. The blood tests indicated the worst: most likely Gustavo had obstructive jaundice. All opinions favored taking him to Hospital Infantil de México (Hospital Infantil), the oldest and, at that time, most prestigious children's hospital in Mexico, where there was a surgeon who had experience with this condition. The director of that hospital, Dr. Lazaro Benavides, was a professor of mine and was kind enough to solicit the chief of

---

4 Conditions of the blood, blood clotting mechanisms and blood-forming tissues.

5 Disease affecting the liver.

6 Jaundice resulting from obstruction of the flow of bile from the liver.

7 Tubes that carry bile (fluid made by the liver, stored in the gallbladder and helps the body digest fats).

8 Surgical re-connection of the ends of bile ducts to intestine, in this case.

surgery and the chief of infectious diseases to see my son.

I was dismayed that these two prominent doctors did not even examine Gustavo. They just looked at him from afar, they looked at the laboratory results and then they started a dialogue between themselves in English, assuming we could not understand what they were discussing. They said it was quite obvious that the baby had biliary atresia and that he should have an operation. The consultation was brief—it all happened standing up. I did not even have the opportunity to look into the surgeon's eyes. He would not look at me and did not even offer his hand to shake. The surgeon said that he could do the operation the following Monday. We had no choice but to accept his offer. For this surgeon, it seemed that Gustavo was just another case and the operation would be just another operation. For my family, however, these events were the most painful of our lives. We felt very lonely.

This is how I learned that for surgeons who operate everyday, an operation scheduled tomorrow is just another routine case. For parents, it is an extraordinary, once in a lifetime event in which the life of the person they love most is at stake. That is why they deserve complete reverence and compassion.

To the world you may be one person,

but to one person you might be the world.

—*Anonymous*

*****

Many years later, those images race back to my mind when I observe doctors during an interview, concentrating on their computer screens instead of their patients. I wonder if all this technological "progress" contributes to the passive, impersonal relationship between doctors and patients. It is hard to believe that there are voices suggesting that doctors must try to avoid becoming emotionally involved with their patients. Without the human ingredient and compassion, medicine and surgery would be just another technical activity.

*****

We left the children's hospital feeling devastated. Rosalinda, my wife at the time, was crying, carrying Gustavo in her arms. Standing at the entrance of the hospital was my mentor, Dr. Jesus Lozoya. For political reasons, he rarely went to that hospital but for some mysterious reason, he was there that day. He saw us and asked what brought us to the hospital. While I explained what was happening, he noticed that Rosalinda was crying.

"Alberto, are you happy having your child receive an operation in this institution? If you are not, I will be happy to help you take your son to another country. I have friends in the Soviet Union and the United States. Think about it and come to my house this afternoon."

Later that day, I told Dr. Lozoya that I just finished a book by a doctor from Boston by the name of Robert Gross. "I know that my son's prognosis is not good, Dr. Lozoya. Cases like his carry a very small chance to be the type of defect that could be successfully repaired. But I still want to explore that possibility under the care of Dr. Gross." I had no idea at the time that Dr. Lozoya and Dr. Gross were good friends.

Dr. Lozoya grabbed the phone. "Bob, I have here one of my residents who's baby is ill. There is a possibility that his son has biliary atresia and he wants to travel to Boston for you to operate on him. Yes. Yes, he's aware that there is very little to offer his child, but he still wants to take the opportunity for you to operate...."

After the conversation with Dr. Gross, Dr. Lozoya gave me a check to pay for the tickets to Boston. "Pay me later, Alberto. Whenever you can." Concerning the payment of the hospital, he instructed me to talk to the administrator and request credit so I could pay by installments.

Since I had to cancel the operation at the hospital in Mexico, I phoned the director and explained that I was very grateful for his help but decided to go elsewhere for the procedure. The director advised me to notify the surgeon and let him know my decision directly.

When I spoke to the surgeon I was shocked by his response. He became irate, "I am sure this is a consequence of Dr. Lozoya's influence but I want to tell you that he does not know anything about these conditions."

I explained that I appreciated his offer and knew that the chances for my son were very few but I hoped he would understand that I was going to Boston because I wanted the best for my son. I did not expect his answer, "Yes, I understand what *malinchismo* is all about."

Malinchismo requires an explanation. When Hernan Cortes conquered Mexico, he found that the Aztecs had a powerful empire. The conquest included many bloody battles and thousands of killings. Eventually, Cortes married an Aztec lady called Malinche and had *mestizo* (racially mixed) children with her. Even today, Malinche is a controversial figure in Mexico. For some, she is the symbol of the racial integration that made Mexico what it is now, a symbol of the mix of races, which may be considered the formula for a peaceful future planet. Conversely, others consider Malinche a figure of treason, a collaborationist who contributed to the Spanish conquest of the Aztecs. As a consequence, every time a Mexican shows any kind of preference for foreign technology, foreign articles or imported goods, it is considered *malinchista*—a very pejorative word. When the surgeon called me malinchista, it took me by surprise and I could not answer. I did not have any desire to discuss this further or become part of any controversy. I was young and very concerned about my son.

After that incident, I promised myself never to be offended

when my patients or their parents say things I considered to be inappropriate or when they make decisions that do not agree with me. Surgeons have sensitive egos. Parents sometimes go to other centers for a second or even a third opinion. The discomfort doctors may feel when their knowledge or skill is questioned is slight compared with the anguish and anxiety that parents feel. Confronting the potential death or pain of their precious child, the amount of suffering that parents endure is so enormous that there is no right or reason to be upset with them.

I like to believe that my attitude with my patients' parents has been a key to my professional success. As far as I am concerned, parents can do or tell me whatever they want because they are living an extremely trying situation. I have been there. Today, when a young couple comes to my office with their ailing baby, I look at their faces. I cannot avoid thinking about my time with Gustavo.

*****

We went to Boston. When we arrived at the airport, Ms. Jean Lootz was waiting for us with a car. Assuming that she was Dr. Gross' secretary, we sat in the backseat. We noticed that she wore a large diamond ring and thought that was a little unusual of a secretary. Later at Dr. Gross' home, we learned that Jean was his beloved woman, a magnificent human being and his lifelong companion. Jean and Dr. Gross were not married because, amongst other issues, Dr. Gross' wife would not divorce him.

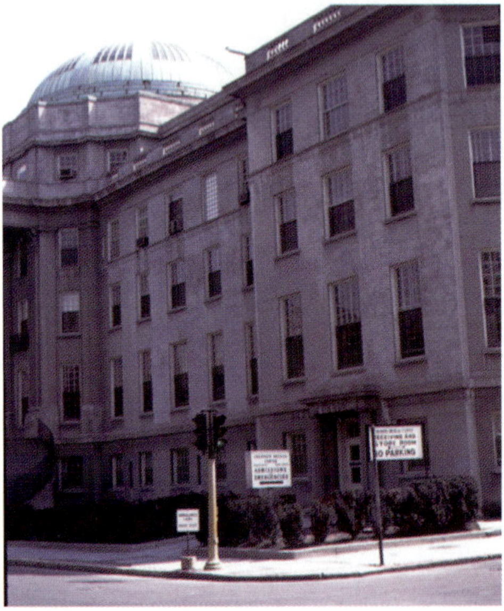

Children's Hospital Medical Center Boston

Jean Lootz took us directly to Children's Hospital Boston. Forty-eight hours later, Gustavo was operated on by Dr. Gross only to find that he had a non-repairable type of biliary atresia. We were devastated. We asked Dr. Gross how long our baby would live and he said about nine months. Gustavo lived almost five years with no further treatment. Those five years were extremely challenging for him and for Rosalinda, who spent most of her time with Gustavo while I was working. Gustavo was a sweet boy with a special, sensitive personality. He was small and fragile, yet he was always protective of his two, big, strong, younger brothers.

It is certainly an excruciating pain for parents to see their baby's misery and not being able to help him. Perhaps, it is even more painful to perceive that the child grows and develops his own personality. He becomes aware of his condition and asks many questions—questions that cannot be answered.

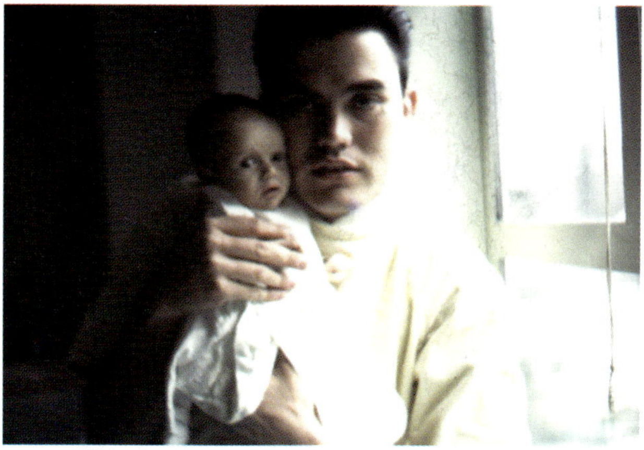

With Gustavo at Children's Hospital Boston

During his short life, Gustavo endured several episodes of pneumonia, serious episodes of bleeding due to coagulation disorders,[9] irritability from the increased bilirubin in his blood and tissues, and two fractures due to fragile bones. During that time, we met extraordinary doctors who helped with exemplary professionalism. Regrettably, we also met others not worth remembering.

*****

During the 10 days that we were in Boston, Dr. Gross and Jean Lootz were very gracious and generous. They invited us for dinner

9 Disorders with the body's ability to control blood clotting.

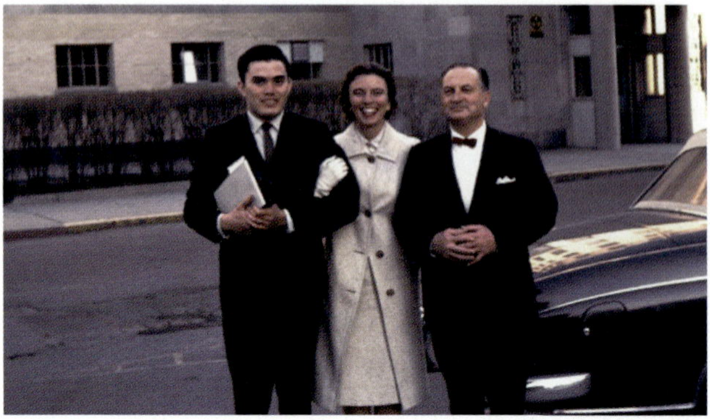

Left to right: Alberto Peña, Jean Lootz, Robert Gross
Boston 1965

at elegant restaurants and to their home for the weekend. During our conversations we learned more about the old friendship between Dr. Lozoya and Dr. Gross. On Sunday, we attended the local Baptist church, which was Rosalinda's religion. There, the minister was a young man by the name of Victor Scalise. We sat in the back and when Victor finished his sermon he came directly to us.

"You are new here, right? Where are you from?"

"We are from Mexico."

"Mexico? What are you doing here?"

We explained the reason for our visit and told him that we were staying in a rented room near the hospital. "You don't have to be there. You are coming with me to my home." Victor took us to get our baggage and we went to his house. During an entire week, Victor and Mary, his loving wife, were very gracious and generous. A great friendship was born and has lasted until now.

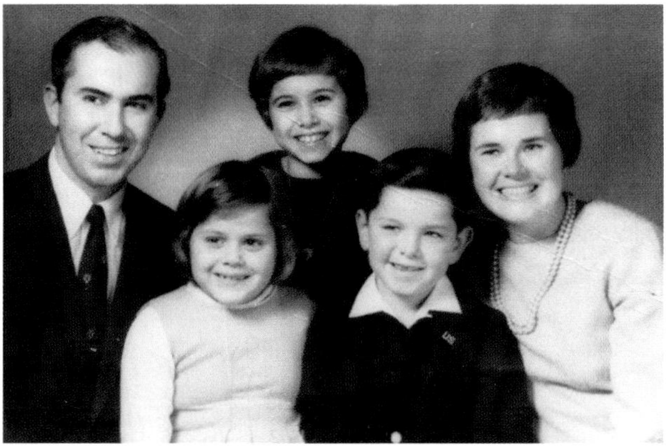

Victor and Mary Scalise
Children: Caroline, Suzanne and Douglas

At the end of our time in Boston, Victor Scalise handed me a check, "The members of my church want you to have this."

"But, Victor, I am not Baptist."

"I know. But this is a present for you both."

*****

The night before we left Boston, I met once more with Dr. Gross. "Please, let me talk to the administration. I want to ask about the bill and I need your help to get credit so that I can pay by installments."

Dr. Gross replied, "There is no bill. Everything has been taken care of."

I still do not know what happened. I suppose Dr. Gross paid the bill or arranged with the administration so that they did not charge me a cent. We actually returned to Mexico City with more money than the little that we had in our pockets when we left. Of course, Rosalinda and I were very distraught because of the terrible news about our baby, but the whole trip had been such an amazingly positive human experience that it gave us hope—a hope that has reverberated through the rest of my life.

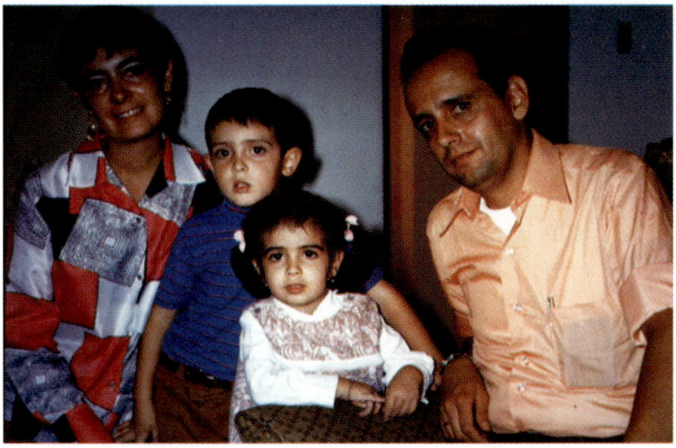

A great friend Dr. Manuel Pintos, his wife Barbara, Emanuel and Barbara Jr.

As soon as I arrived in Mexico City, I went to Dr. Lozoya to thank him and tell him about the trip. I inquired about the terms to pay him by monthly installments out of my meager salary. Dr. Lozoya replied, "There is no need to pay anything. Dr. Manuel Pintos was here and took care of everything." Manuel Pintos is one of my dear friends. At that time he was an intern and had a very meager salary. This is a reason I like to repeat:

Brothers are the friends we did not select
and friends are the brothers we selected.

*****

Against the prognosis dictated by most statistics, Gustavo actually lived 4½ years. We tried to avoid his suffering as much as possible. My first decision was to try to keep him away from hospitals. Medical treatments, including blood transfusions, were given at home. A few days before Christmas in 1969, Gustavo had bronchopneumonia and severe respiratory distress, he heard me talking about the possibility of taking him to the hospital. I was holding him in my arms when he said his last words, "Do not take me to the hospital." Very few experiences in life can be as painfully profound as watching the death of a son.

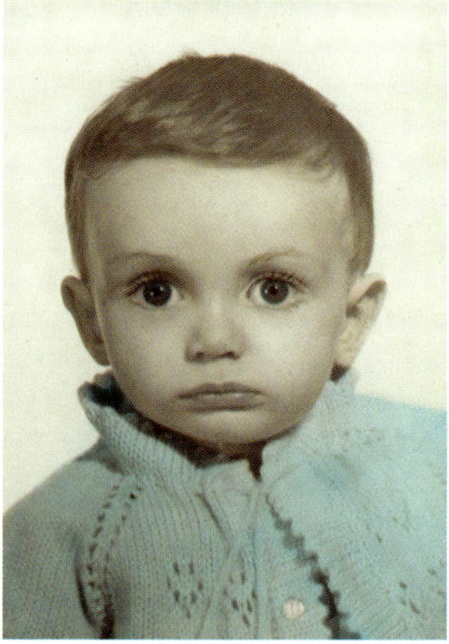

Gustavo

When my son died, liver transplants were considered experimental. If Gustavo were born today he would be a candidate for a transplant. I cannot stop thinking what would be better—being born in 1965 and dying young or being born in 2010, enduring the trials of being on the list of transplant recipients (with high chances of dying while waiting), having a liver transplant (with the risk of dying) and a life full of constant medical supervision (always at risk of a rejection). I have no clear answers for those questions but I feel at peace with the way things happened. With everything that occurred at a sensitive stage in my professional life, Gustavo's short life influenced me in an extremely positive way. He will always be a major factor to explain my career.

THOSE WHO INFLUENCED ME MOST

Like anyone else, I was deeply influenced by my parents. My father was an agronomist, my mother a housewife. She was 16 and he was 25 when they got married. They had eight children, but three died; the oldest from typhoid fever, the second from gastroenteritis and the third from respiratory infection. Their marriage lasted for 15 years and they divorced when I was five years old. I have reasons to believe that my parents had problems even before I was born. My father wanted to call me Alberto, which was his brother's name but my mother wanted to call me Gustavo, which was her father's and brother's names. My mother believed that Catholic baptism was very important but my father believed that the official government registration was more important than the baptism. Consequently, my father took me to the government office and registered me with the name of Alberto. My mother ignored that and took me to the Catholic Church and baptized me with the name of Gustavo!

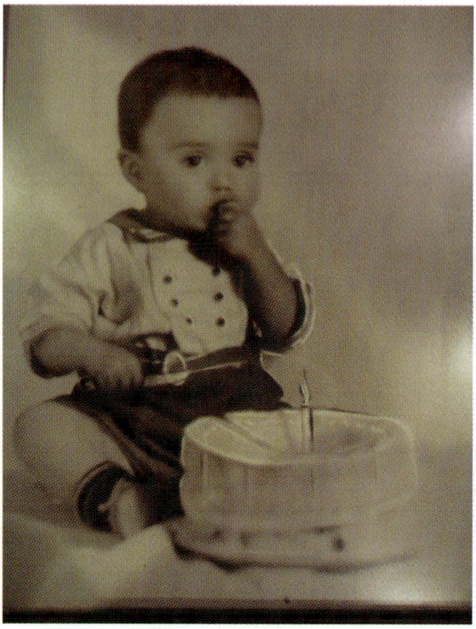
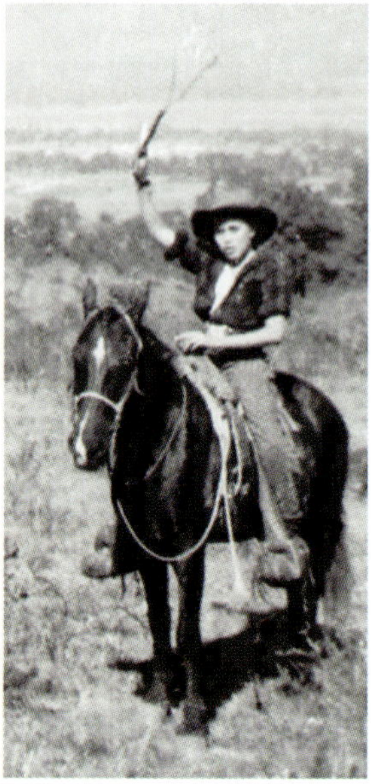

Left: One year old; Right: 12 years old "Mexican Revolutionary"

After they divorced, what followed was a stressful and certainly not boring life. My siblings and I had a tough time. The divorce divided us; two children (including me) stayed with my mother, the other three with my father. It was painful. During the six years of my primary education, I passed through nine different schools with the name Gustavo and only finished one full year. Due to complicated circumstances we were changing addresses and cities. In order for me to obtain my elementary school certificate, my mother left me with an aunt for several months.

When my mother registered me in secondary school, the school authorities requested to see my birth certificate and inquired why it read Alberto while my elementary school certificate read Gustavo.

She explained to them that my name was actually Gustavo-Alberto. Because of that, my high school certificate reads Gustavo-Alberto. At the university, though, they insisted that the name Alberto should appear first because that was the name on my birth certificate. Consequently, my university certificate reads Alberto-Gustavo.

The real crisis occurred when I applied to Escuela Médico Militar (Military Medical School). There was a very serious captain in charge of registering all the candidates. He had the stereotypical boisterous military tone to his voice and a very short temper:

"Sir, you are presenting three certificates with three different names *and* a birth certificate with another name. Can you explain to me what in the hell are you trying to pull here? Who are you, goddamnit?"

I adjusted myself, tried to sound friendly and polite, and explained to the captain the peculiar origin of my name. While doing so, many applicants lined up behind me and made fun of me. The captain must have been moved by my story because he did not make any more comments but simply sealed several papers with my now official name: Alberto. This event was eventually revealed to my whole family and it offended some members of my mother's family. They were angry because they thought that I was the one that changed my family given name, Gustavo.

In spite of all of these problems, both of my parents were always very loving, regardless of their personal conflicts. Perhaps, the most important component of their influence was that my mother and father always supported their children. They both believed that we would achieve many things in the future. Fortunately, they lived long lives and were able to see their children grow to have happy, rewarding and productive lives.

*****

I decided to study medicine and chose the Military Medical School in Mexico City primarily because it had a great reputation for being very selective, disciplined and academically superior. Because of its selection, the number of students was limited, making the opportunities to learn and practice even better. More importantly, it was free. It was not easy to be admitted, but once accepted, one could spend six years studying medicine, receiving uniforms, food (not very good, but free) and a room. Additionally, the school was located next to a great 700 bed teaching general hospital. No question, it was a great school. I feel an enormous gratitude towards my Alma Mater and the Mexican army for what I learned and received.

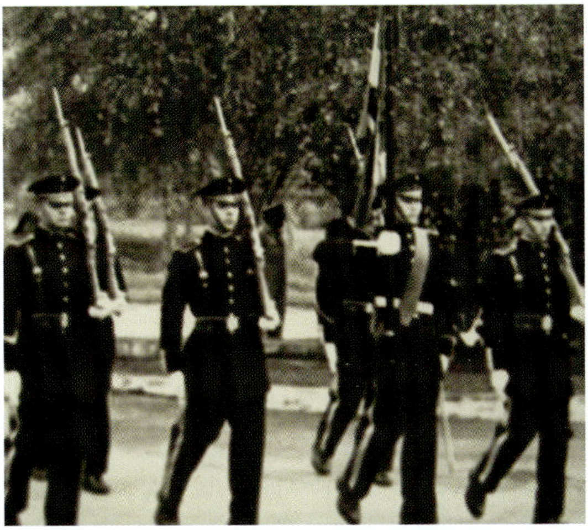

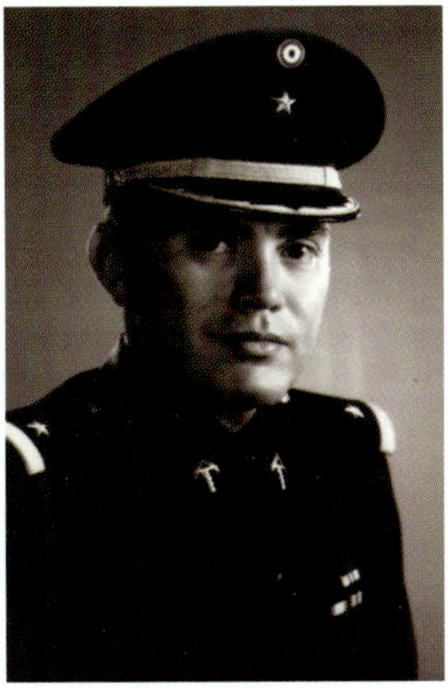

Left: Military Medical School (Mexico) Carrying the flag; Right: Graduated Military Medical School; Below: Military hospital renovated

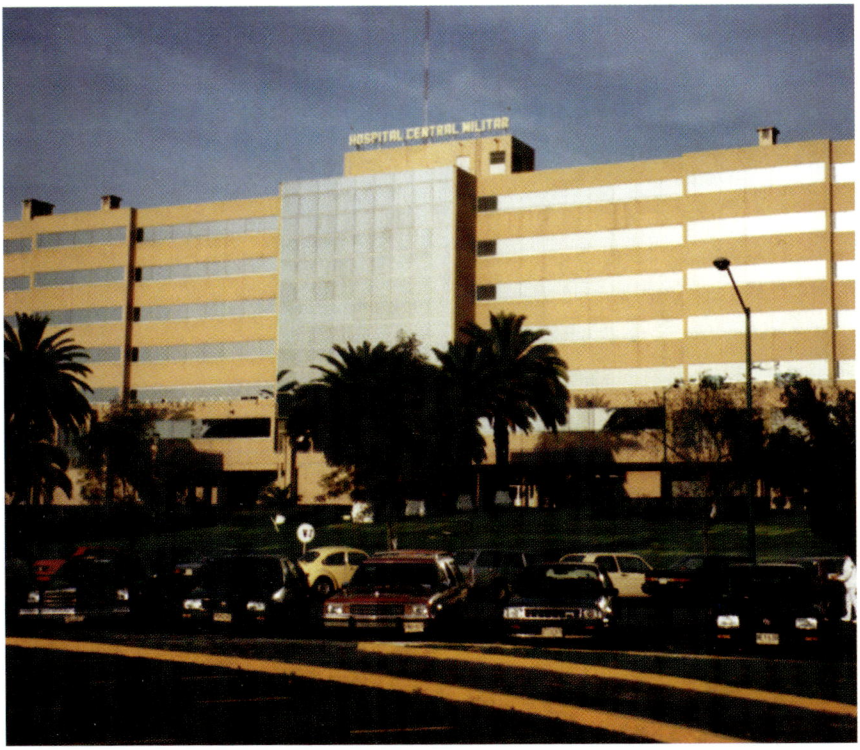

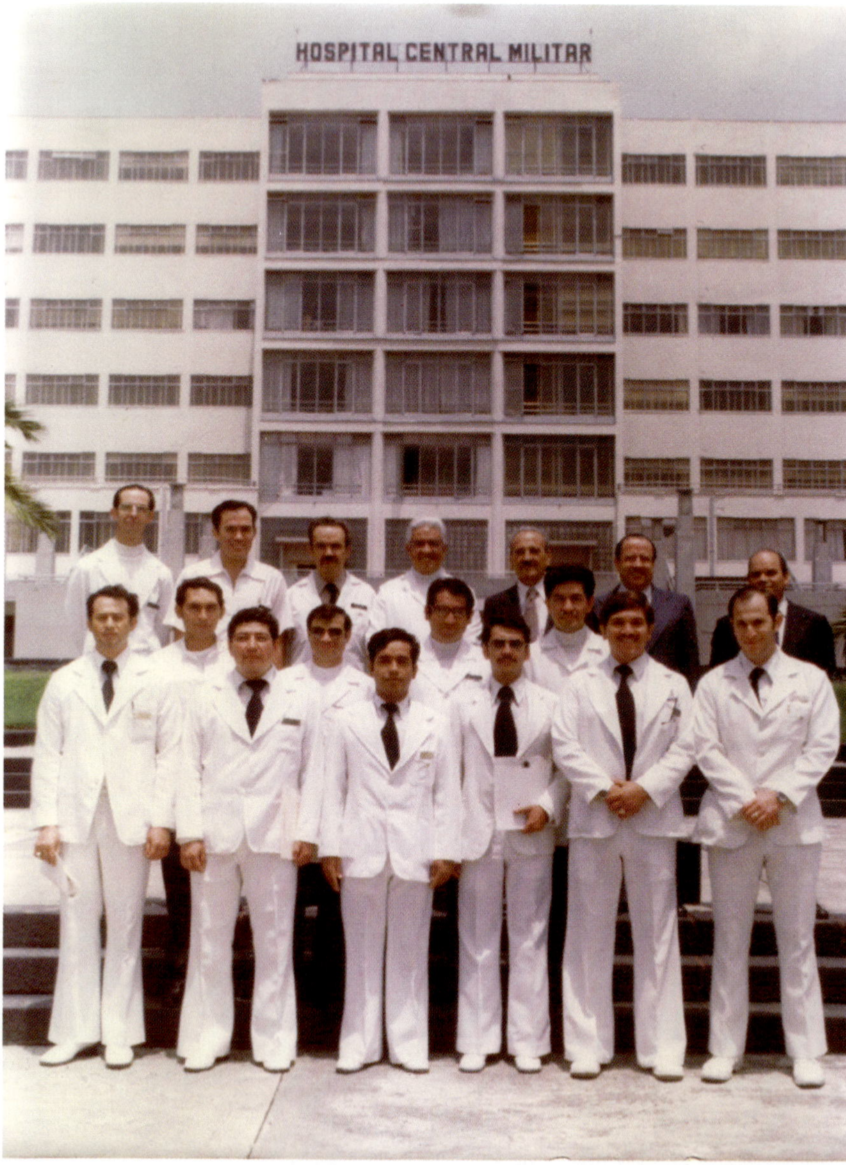

Military Hospital Pediatric Staff
Back row from left to right: Luis Limón, Alberto Peña, Juan Avila-Marcué, Daniel Rolón, Jesus Lozoya, Alberto Amor, Unidentified;
Front row from left to right: Unidentified, Octavio Martinez-Natera, Unidentified, Juan de la Fuente, Unidentified, Rolando Cuevas, Unidentified, José Arizmendi, Unidentified, Unidentified

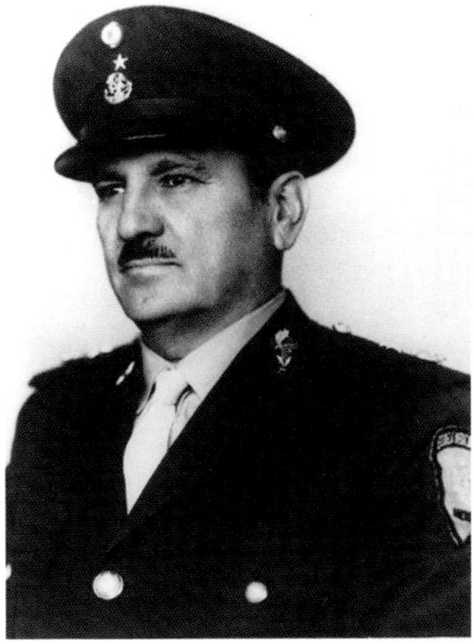

DR. JESUS LOZOYA

Pediatrics was taught during the last year of school. The professor of the course was Dr. Jesus Lozoya—certainly, a very impressive man. Dr. Lozoya also had a rather humble origin, born in the state of Chihuahua. He was a military doctor and in 1938, when he was a young pediatrician, he managed to obtain a scholarship to continue his training in pediatrics at Case Western Reserve Hospital in Cleveland, Ohio. However, he was very interested in what was happening in the field of pediatric surgery, more specifically, he was interested in what Dr. William Ladd was doing in Boston.

Children's Hospital Boston is where pediatric surgery began in the United States and flourished due to the hard work of its pioneer: Dr. William Ladd. Dr. Lozoya requested an extension of his license from the Mexican army to continue his trip at Children's

Hospital Boston for a few more months. I do not know exactly how many months Dr. Lozoya spent in Boston or exactly what kind of activity he had in Dr. Ladd's service but he became well-known by him. Around this time is when he met and became a good friend of one of Dr. Ladd's collaborators, Dr. Robert E. Gross. Subsequently, Dr. Lozoya was one of the members of a selected group of pediatric surgeons that created the Surgical Section of the American Academy of Pediatrics together with Doctors William Ladd, Robert Gross, Everett Koop (former Surgeon General of the United States) amongst others. (Ref. 2)

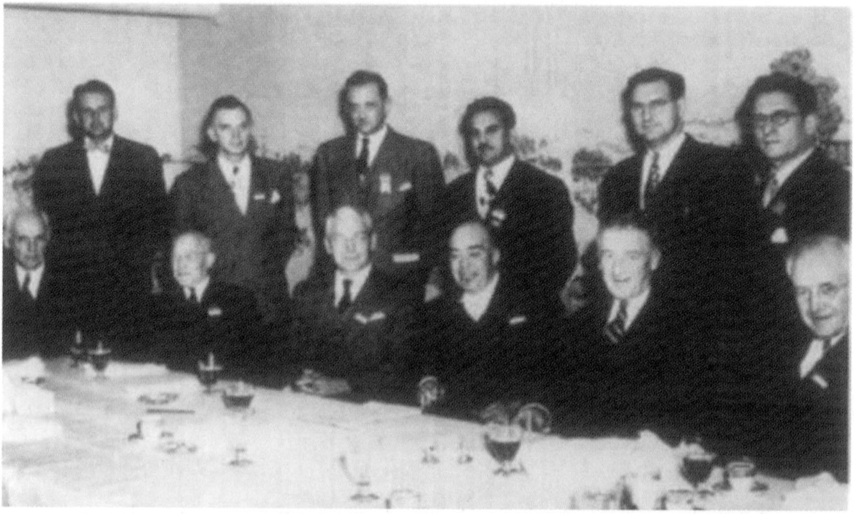

First meeting of the Section of Surgery of the AAP, Haddon-Chalfont Hotel, Atlantic City, November 21, 1948; Seated left to right: Doctors Ladd, Coe, Ingraham, Wyatt, Lanman, and Sweet; Standing left to right: Doctors Swan, Bowman, Potts, Lozoya, Koop, and Fontana from Uruguay

Dr. Lozoya returned to Mexico when the president (a general), influenced by another famous Mexican military pediatrician, Dr. Federico Gomez (considered the pioneer of pediatrics in Mexico), constructed the first children's hospital in the country. Dr. Lozoya was one of its founders, becoming the first chief of surgery of the brand new Hospital Infantil from 1943 until 1951.

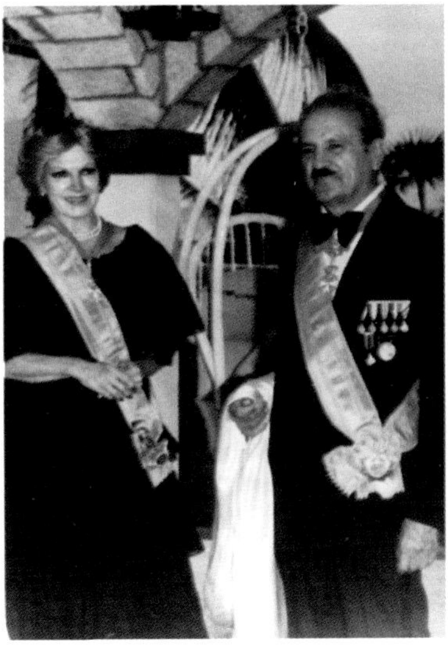

Margarita and Jesus Lozoya

Dr. Lozoya was an extremely intelligent, ambitious, entrepreneur and politically oriented person. During those years, he managed to have a very large, private clinical practice. He continued serving in the army and became a general. He was also a very distinguished politician and was elected senator and governor of his native state of Chihuahua. He also owned a pharmaceutical laboratory and became a very prosperous businessman. Dr. Lozoya was a great speaker. He spent much of his time organizing associations, federations and confederations of pediatrics in Mexico. In addition to the Surgical Section of the American Academy of Pediatrics, he was one of the founders of the Pacific Association of Pediatric

Surgeons and what now is known as the World Federation of Associations of Pediatric Surgeons. That is why his time dedicated to pediatric surgery was rather short. Dr. Lozoya and Dr. Federico Gomez (director of Hospital Infantil) did not get along well and in 1951 Dr. Lozoya left that institution and worked exclusively at the Hospital Central Militar (Central Military Hospital). There, he was professor of pediatrics and chief of the department (including pediatric surgery).

I met Dr. Lozoya in 1961, during my last year of medical school. As a student, I liked Dr. Lozoya very much: he was very charismatic, his presentations were brilliant and a little folkloric, and that made him all the more interesting. It was delightful to be in his class. A couple of years before, Dr. Lozoya suffered the loss of one of his children in a fatal car accident. That young man happened to be a medical student at Universidad Nacional Autonoma de México; so, to honor his son, Dr. Lozoya created an award that he gave to the best student of his class every year. The medal was named for his son: Jesus Lozoya-Thalmann. That particular year, Dr. Lozoya decided that I would receive the Jesus Lozoya-Thalmann prize! When I received the medal from Dr. Lozoya, I confided in him that I wanted to be a pediatric surgeon. From day one, he supported me in every way he could.

Dr. Lozoya firmly believed that in order to be a pediatric surgeon, a doctor should be a pediatrician first (like he was), learning everything about the anatomy and physiology of a child and *then* make a decision about what path to follow. To become a pediatric surgeon, the young pediatrician was supposed to continue training for three extra years. In other words, in Mexico, it was not a requirement to be trained in general surgery to become a pediatric surgeon. Dr. Lozoya created this particular method of training and it is still employed in some Latin American countries today.

In the United States, on the other hand, pediatric surgery was founded and created by surgeons; so, only those who were fully trained as surgeons could apply for a fellowship in pediatric surgery. I supported the idea of learning general surgery before getting into pediatric surgical training. Dr. Lozoya and I had many heated discussions about the subject and never came to an agreement on that matter. As a consequence of his persistence, I trained in both pediatrics *and* general surgery before training in pediatric surgery. My training lasted for a total of nine years. Three of them were spent in Boston.

When I finished medical school, I continued my internship and residency at the Central Military Hospital in Mexico City where I was trained in general surgery. During my residency, I demonstrated a special interest in pediatric surgical cases and became very familiar with the staff in the department. I actually did not learn much pediatric surgery from Dr. Lozoya. He was a very busy person doing other extra-medical activities and it was not very common to see him in the operating room. However, he and I developed a very good relationship and every time there was an opportunity we had long philosophical conversations. I always had the feeling that, in a way, I was filling the empty space left by his deceased son. Dr. Lozoya became a paternal figure for me as well. His experiences as a doctor, politician, member of the Mexican military and businessman were extremely valuable and guided me through my life. He grew up in a difficult period in Mexico, during the time of revolution and as a result, he developed a particular talent to survive and succeed under adverse circumstances. I learned many non-surgical lessons from Dr. Lozoya. He was a very intuitive man and knew how to obtain the very best from every human being. He was very generous with his time for me; I could call on him whenever I needed. He seemed to enjoy talking to me.

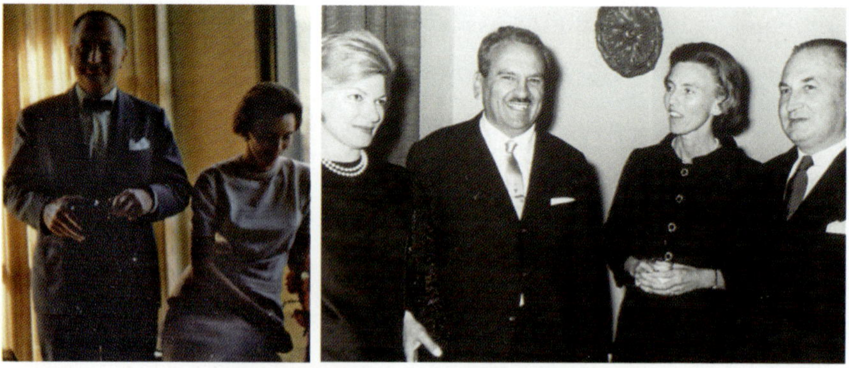

Left: Dr. Gross and Jean, Mexico City, 1968;
Right: Dr. Lozoya & Margarita and Dr. Gross & Jean Lootz

One night, a baby arrived at the Central Military Hospital with an intussusception.[10] Dr. Lozoya used to give an excellent talk about intussusception in his class so I decided to call him at home. A lady answered. I asked her if I had reached Dr. Lozoya's home and if

10 Enfolding of one segment of the intestine within another.

I could speak with him. The lady replied, "This *is* Dr. Lozoya's house but Dr. Lozoya does not live here." Later, I learned that Dr. Lozoya was separated from his wife. She refused to divorce him and therefore, he had been living for several years with Margarita, a wonderful lady who was his companion until he died. I also learned that not only were Dr. Lozoya and Dr. Gross great friends but it seemed that their living arrangements were quite similar. Dr. Lozoya, Margarita, Dr. Gross and Jean Lootz even enjoyed spending Christmas together on Cozumel (at that time, a small and less traveled Mexican island) at a little hotel where Dr. Lozoya had good friends. Every night at dinner, overlooking the Caribbean, Dr. Gross asked the musicians to play a beautiful Mexican song called "El Pájaro Azul" ("The Blue Bird").

*****

Dr. Lozoya and I used to have heated debates about different subjects. Once, during one of these discussions, I complained about some problem and said that I was frustrated. I did not expect Dr. Lozoya's reaction. He was extremely upset and prohibited me to use that word in his presence. He advised me to delete that word from my vocabulary. "Only losers need that word. Frustration is equivalent to a temper tantrum in a spoiled child." After that, I have never felt frustrated again.

Whenever I used to ask Dr. Lozoya for advice, his characteristic answer was: "Do you want me to tell you the truth, Alberto? Or do you want me to rub your back?" I always wanted to know the truth. Thus, what followed was a long, tough, expletive-laden speech that was hard to swallow but extremely important for the formative years of a young doctor.

Many years later, near the end of his life, he asked me for advice. "So," I replied, "Do you want me to tell you the truth? Or do you want me to rub your back?"

His response was not particularly sweet. Most of the words he used are not to be repeated. "You're not supposed to use what I taught you against me, Alberto." We both smiled and laughed at the exchange.

Dr. Lozoya was the person from whom I received the most significant help at a time when my family and I needed it most. Now I know, that for a young person, it is integral to perceive that somebody trusts in him. Dr. Lozoya trusted and supported me at that crucial stage of my life.

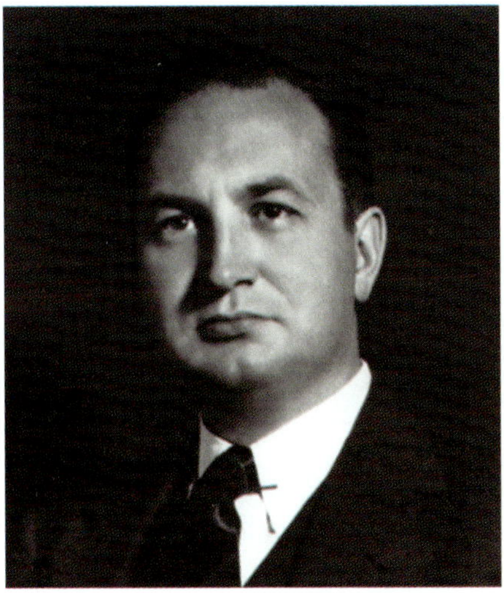

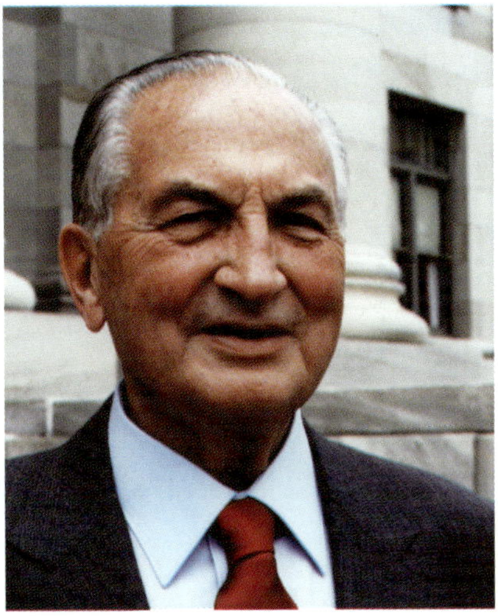

DR. ROBERT E. GROSS

Dr. Gross certainly had a tremendous influence on my professional and personal life. I met him for the first time through Dr. Lozoya in 1965, when he operated on my son, Gustavo. During the days that my son was at Children's Hospital Boston, I asked Dr. Gross if I could watch him doing other operations. He graciously granted me that wish and I was able to observe him for the first time for an entire day, doing open-heart operations as well as general surgical procedures. I was deeply impressed.

Four years after Dr. Gross operated on my son, I decided to look for further training. Dr. Lozoya and I had a long talk about this. I had previously studied and passed the Educational Commission for Foreign Medical Graduates examination and as a result, I could apply to a five-year general surgical training program and be eligible for a position as a fellow in pediatric surgery for two more years. I wanted to retire from the military and receive full training in pediatric surgery in the United States. Dr. Lozoya was adamantly opposed to the idea. He insisted that if I went to the United States for seven years I would never return to Mexico. In retrospect, perhaps he was right. He suggested that I go for a much shorter period of time because I was, in a way, already trained. He said that I just required a short time abroad to become a good pediatric surgeon in Mexico.

After three long hours of talk and negotiations, we agreed that I would go to the United States for three years. Dr. Lozoya was also against the idea of me leaving the army, so he offered to obtain a three year license from the secretary of defense to receive my meager salary as a major (while in the US), with an obligation to return to work for six years as a pediatric surgeon at Central Military Hospital in Mexico City. At that time, I had a sick child who was already four years old, a second son, fortunately very healthy and a third one on the way. So, I accepted Dr. Lozoya's offer and with his help again, I contacted Dr. Gross asking for a position to obtain training at Children's Hospital Boston. He accepted me as a research fellow at his cardiovascular surgical laboratory. Dr. Gross explained that he was no longer chief of general pediatric surgery but took over as chief of cardiac surgery. He told me that I could stay at his laboratory for one year only and after that I had to look for another place. I graciously accepted Dr. Gross' offer as a research fellow for one year. In the back of mind, though, I was a bit concerned about what would I do in the United States for the remaining two years of my army license when this yearlong fellowship ended.

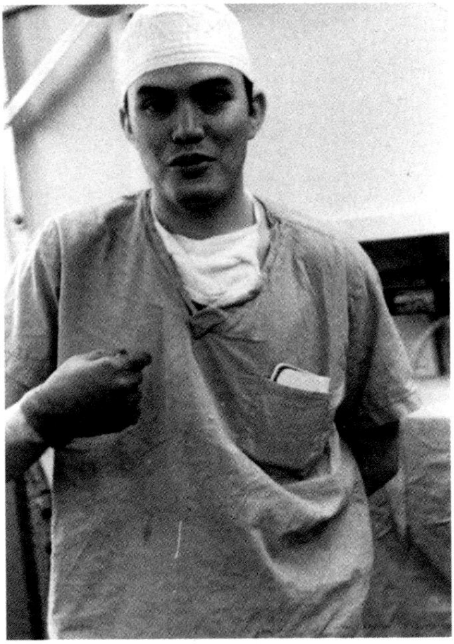

Dr. Peña, Research Fellow
Boston, 1969

DR. GROSS' LABORATORY

My family and I returned to Boston in the winter of January 1969. My first assignment at Children's Hospital Boston was to work at Dr. Gross' laboratory with Dr. Jimmy Jones and Dr. Bert Litwin.

With Dr. Jones, I assisted in lung re-implantations in dogs as a preliminary step to lung transplantation—a wonderful experience from a technical point of view. A few months into this assignment, feeling more adjusted to my surroundings, Dr. Jones came to me,

"Alberto, I am inviting you to a moving party on Sunday. There will be plenty of food and drinks. Will you come?"

I was new, he was my chief and so I was not brave enough to ask if I could bring my family, particularly because the invitation was for a Sunday (a day most dedicate to family). I showed up on time to Jimmy Jones' house to enjoy the "moving party." I was under the impression that there would be an orchestra and dancing to promote the "moving" part of the event. I was very disappointed to find that I had actually been recruited to help Jimmy move to another house. From 10 a.m. to 5 p.m., we transported all of his family belongings from one house to another. After that, I became more inquisitive about the nature of the parties that I was invited to in the United States. Jimmy is a wonderful person and we remain in contact.

With Dr. Bert Litwin, we created aortic pulmonary shunts[11] in dogs, which at that time was a palliative procedure[12] done in newborns (the so-called "blue babies") with a complex cardiac condition known as tetralogy of Fallot. A submarine-like operating room located in the sub-basement of Children's Hospital Boston, the hyperbaric chamber was very active in caring for patients with gas gangrene[13] as well as very sick newborn babies with cardiac conditions requiring palliative procedures. Already very

---

11 Surgically created passage (anastomosis) between the aorta and pulmonary artery.

12 Relief of the symptoms of a disease or disorder without a cure. A temporary fix.

13 Form of gangrene occurring in a wound infected with anaerobic bacteria and characterized by the presence of gas in the affected tissue.

sick newborn babies could not tolerate major surgery but the hyperbaric chamber allowed us to perform operations under a three-atmosphere pressure, improving oxygenation in the babies, helping them to survive. Although the operations did not repair the malformation completely, they aimed to allow those unfortunate children to survive and reach the age required to tolerate a full, open-heart repair.

Dr. Bert Litwin was an excellent technical surgeon. From him, I learned delicate tissue handling and meticulous techniques: We were making two to three millimeter shunts between the pulmonary artery and aorta in dogs to determine the optimal size shunt that could be constructed in humans, ultimately improving oxygenation. Every time one of the surgical residents could not tolerate the pressure in the chamber, I was there, waiting in the middle of the night, ready to scrub-in with Dr. Litwin.

All that was very interesting; however, my passion was always in caring for children. Everyday, when I finished my work in the laboratory, I ran to the main operating rooms of the hospital to watch Doctors Robert Filler, Arnold Colodny, Samuel Schuster, Kenneth Welch and Angelo Eraklis perform different surgical procedures in children.

From my first day at Children's Hospital Boston, I told Dr. Judah Folkman (the chief of Surgery) and Dr. Robert Filler (responsible for the clinical training program) that I wanted to have an opportunity to work clinically with patients. They explained that clinical training positions were given with years of anticipation and it would be nearly impossible for me to have an opportunity.

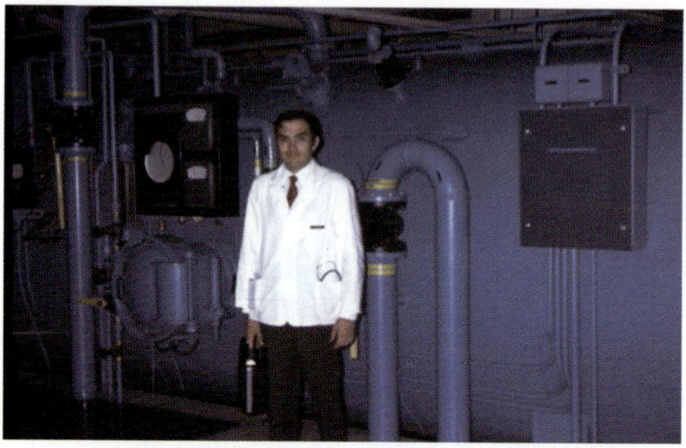

**Dr. Peña, Senior Resident, hyperbaric chamber
Boston, 1971**

UNFORESEEN INFLUENCE

After a few months of working in Dr. Gross' laboratory, I sent letters to many American children's hospitals in preparation for my move after my contract as a research fellow ended. This is when the serendipitous part of my life began. As a consequence of the Vietnam War, the United States was recruiting surgeons to be sent to the frontline and some of the residents from the Peter Bent Brigham Hospital were drafted. In those years, the surgical residents from Peter Bent Brigham Hospital rotated for one year as junior residents at Children's Hospital Boston. One of the residents was drafted, leaving a one-year opening for a junior resident. Dr. Filler generously offered me the job and I accepted. I do not know how much influence Dr. Gross had in this matter but I was very happy, nonetheless. I had not even finished the one-year of research fellowship when I became a surgical junior resident. As it turned out, this came when I had been working for only nine months. Dr. Filler explained that this prospect was only for one year and he could not promise anything for the future. For me, it was a great opportunity; I had great enthusiasm and prepared myself to learn as much as possible during that year.

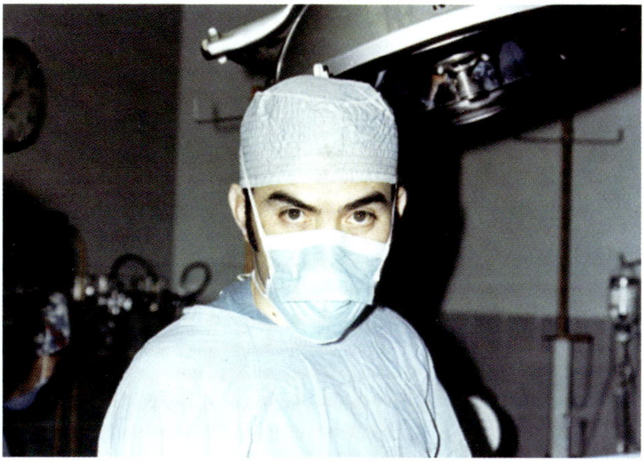

Dr. Peña, Junior Surgical Resident
Boston, 1970

But tragedy struck. Gustavo died at home 11 months after we arrived in Boston in 1969. It was a difficult time; however, as parents we felt that Gustavo's life was torture and he deserved rest and peace. Again, as painful as it was, we did not feel alone. Although our families were in Mexico, we had great friends in Victor and Mary Scalise and Dr. Gross and Jean Lootz. There are not enough words to express the gratitude they generated in our hearts.

Time moved on and I still had to figure out what to do with my third year in the United States. Once more, I sent letters to several

American children's hospitals. Then, something exceptionally rare occurred. One of the official pediatric surgery fellows at Children's Hospital Boston got sick. He was not feeling well, had a chest x-ray done and found that he had a tuberculosis cavity on one of his lungs. He was forced to leave the program to care for himself. He had only been a fellow for ten months and there were 14 more months that remained to complete his two-year training program. Amazingly, I also had 14 months left in my army permission. Serendipity again! I was there in the right place at the right time and I replaced that unfortunate young surgeon. Those 14 months were extremely productive and crucial in my training.

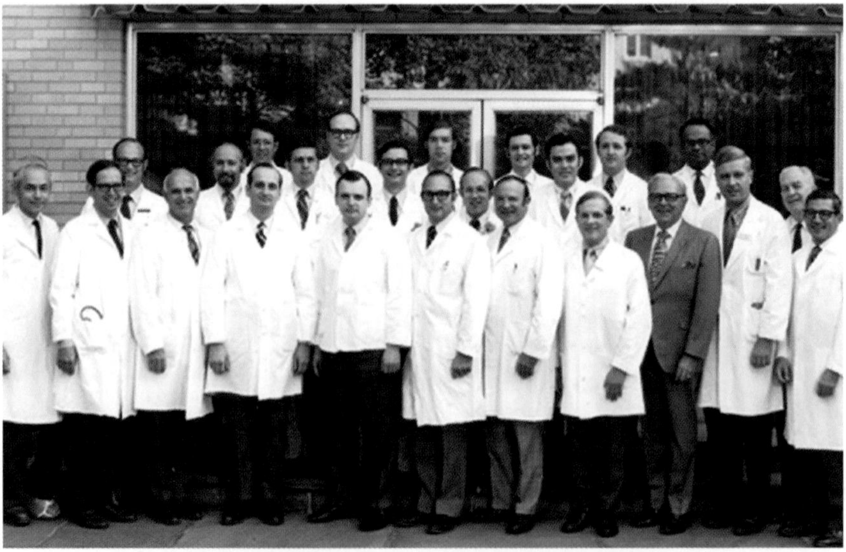

1971 Surgical Staff, Children's Hospital Boston
Left to right front row: Arnold Colodny, Ray Levy, Joseph Murray (Nobel Prize), Judah Folkman, Willis Williams, Robert Filler, Kenneth Welch, Samuel Schuster, Donald McCollum, John Gifford, Angelo Eraklis
Left to right back row: Arvin Phillipart, Allan Perlmutter, Michael Mitchell, Mutaz Habal, Michael Meguid, Unidentitified, Unidentitified, Hilleil Laks, Alberto Peña, Bill Cromie, John Daz, John Chamberlain

Certainly, I recognize that I have been extremely fortunate in my life. But, I also learned something widely known: If a person desires something very deeply and believes that it will happen, it may or may not happen. On the contrary, if a person does not believe that that something will happen, it will certainly not happen. Because of this, I am always enthusiastic with young doctors and suggest that they embrace every project and activity with passion and faith. Believe in yourself!

A SERIOUS MAN

Dr. Gross was considered a very serious, almost feared man. If asked, "Is *he* here?" or "Did *he* arrive?" everybody knew that *he* signified Dr. Gross. He usually spoke only a few words. When he felt, for instance, that a resident had dirty shoes, he would tell his secretary to advise the resident to clean them. He was obsessed with everyone having impeccably white shoes. Soon after I became a resident, his secretary called me and gave me a pair of new white shoes for the operating room and instructed me to keep them very clean.

One day, Dr. Gross personally ordered me to come to the hospital the next morning, looking very clean and neat. He did not explain more. I went home a little worried, not knowing exactly what he meant; yet, I was sure that my hair was cut, my fingernails were trimmed and my white uniform was spotless. The next morning, I received a call from the administrator of the hospital and was asked to be present in the director's office. There, they gave me the George von L. Meyer Award, "established to help talented doctors defray the cost of medical education." I am sure Dr. Gross had something to do with that.

*****

In the United States, it is extremely unusual to find people with the name of Jesus; in Mexico, it is very common. One occasion, Dr. Jesus Lozoya visited Dr. Robert Gross at Children's Boston. While in the operating room a surgeon, searching everywhere for Dr. Lozoya, opened the door and asked, "Is Jesus here?" One of the residents answered, "No, Jesus went to have dinner with God." On that night, "God" was none other than Dr. Robert Gross.

*****

In those years at Children's Boston, the two-year training in pediatric surgery included six months rotation in pediatric cardiovascular surgery with Dr. Gross. Even if one was not going to be a cardiac surgeon, many important things were obtained that were enormously useful in practice. Little by little, the resident became more and more active. By the end of the rotation Dr. Gross allowed each of us to do a major cardiovascular operation. The volume of cases was such that it was easy to learn everyday, more and more about specific cardiac operations.

After assisting Dr. Gross in many cases, he allowed me to do a patent ductus arteriosus[14] and then, unbelievably, he allowed me to repair an atrial septal defect![15] Both cases are cardiovascular defects that are now considered relatively simple to correct, but not in those years. Dr. Gross had a perfectly synchronized team that included his scrub nurse[16] and the pump technician[17] (which happened to be his beloved, Jean Lootz). This is why it was not demanding for an amateur like myself to do an open-heart procedure. Actually, his team made things extremely easy, making me feel that I performed the operation. As expected, my lack of experience brought some abrupt misadventures to the procedure. I even heard Dr. Gross exclaim, "Jesus! Jesus!" I still ask myself if he was referring to Jesus Christ or to Dr. Jesus Lozoya for having sent him such an awkward young surgeon.

A MEXICAN CHRISTMAS IN BOSTON

In Mexico, during Christmas, it is common to visit relatives and members of the extended family. In the United States, on the

14 Heart defect that occurs when the temporary fetal blood vessel that connects the aorta and the pulmonary artery does not close at birth. See page 41.

15 Abnormal opening in the wall separating the left and right upper chambers (atria) of the heart.

16 Person that directly hands instruments to the surgeon in the operating room.

17 Person in charge of operating the pump and oxygenator necessary to perform open-heart surgeries.

contrary, most families stay home. It was my family's first Christmas in Boston and we wanted to visit Dr. Gross and Jean who were two of the most important friends that we had in Boston. We hesitated because we heard that in the United States you do not casually show up to a friend's house on Christmas without calling first. I decided, that as a Mexican, I was justified to go with my family to visit Dr. Gross and Jean.

It was in the middle of a snowstorm. Dr. Gross lived in a beautiful house located on the top of a hill on a big piece of land. There was no way for our car to go all the way up the hill to his house. We called from the entrance and Dr. Gross instructed us to wait downhill for him. He came with a tractor pulling a snow car and hauled us up to his house. To our surprise, he was alone with Jean and they were having a very simple dinner. We said that we just dropped by to wish them a "Merry Christmas" and wanted to go back home where our dinner was waiting. Dr. Gross and Jean did not allow us to leave and insisted we stay.

During my time in Boston, a great friend of mine from medical school, Dr. Manuel Pintos (now an ophthalmologist, poet and musician), sent me a letter requesting a very special favor. He had a good friend, Dr. Giovanni Porras, who happened to be the chief surgical resident at Hospital Infantil. He wanted to give his friend a great surprise on the occasion of his graduation as pediatric surgeon. He wanted to present him with the new *Atlas of Pediatric Surgery* (Ref. 3), recently published by Dr. Gross. Not only would he give him the book but he also wanted it signed and dedicated by Dr. Gross to Dr. Porras.

Could I do that? Manuel Pintos is one of those extraordinary friends to whom I could not say no. He is also the one who volunteered to pay Dr. Lozoya the money that he lent to me to take my first son to Boston. But how could I approach Dr. Gross with a book and ask him to write a few words for a person that he never met?

I waited for a day that I saw Dr. Gross alone in his office and was brave enough to walk in and asked him to write something in the book. He usually wrote only a few words, such as, "With kind regards, Robert E. Gross." He was not very eloquent in his dedications of books. That day, for mysterious reasons, he wrote many nice things for Dr. Porras. I sent the book back to Manuel Pintos and he was able to surprise Giovanni with a gift he appreciated very much.

In return, Dr. Porras, a very sensitive man, decided to write a two-page poem to Dr. Gross. Without even knowing me, he sent me the poem written in Spanish and requested that I translate it and present it to Dr. Gross. There I was, trying to translate a poem full of elegant, sophisticated metaphors and Spanish words into English. A poem dedicated to Dr. Gross by a young Mexican surgeon attempting to transport a little bit of the warm Latin temperament into the Anglo-Saxon, highly technical, efficient environment of Children's Hospital Boston. It took several weeks to do so. Again, I was looking for the opportunity to confront Dr. Gross.

That particular Christmas at his home afforded such an occasion. We were celebrating the holiday: enjoying dinner and a couple of glasses of champagne. I had the poem in my pocket. I thought it was the right time, so I cleared my throat. "Dr. Gross, I have something for you," and I read the poem. Amazingly, he began to cry.

Against general opinions, I always found Dr. Gross to be a warm human being. I wondered if he was particularly warm with us, because of Dr. Lozoya's friendship or because we came from Mexico and were not a part of the political intrigues of the hospital. Later, when I returned to Mexico, my great friend Manuel Pintos introduced me to Dr. Giovanni Porras. The three of us have enjoyed a great friendship all these years.

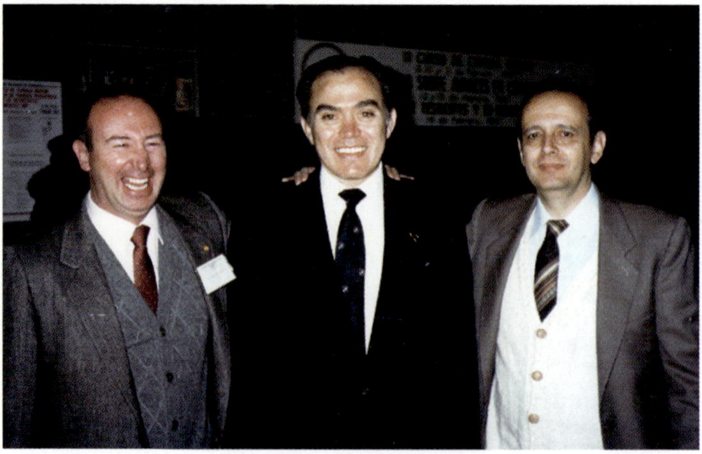

Great friends
Giovanni Porras, Alberto Peña, Manuel Pintos

ANOTHER MAN'S TREASURE

One day, Dr. Gross called me to his office, "Alberto, I have some slides in those big boxes. See if they are useful to you and take them with you."

The boxes were big, metallic and heavy; inside were old glass slides of Dr. Gross's work. These slides were not junk at all. In actuality, he was giving me his entire slide collection and for me, these slides were a treasure! There was only one problem: To view them it was necessary to have an old type of projector that was no longer available. Because I did not have money to take those huge metallic boxes to Mexico, an alternative to the old projector was to copy all the slides into regular 35 mm slides. My great friend, Dr. Willis Williams, proposed a solution to copy all of these slides. Willis is an extraordinarily creative friend. He designed a wooden box where the glass slides could be placed on one side and the camera on the other. It took us about a week, working at night, to copy all of those slides. Many of the slides are still part of my personal collection.

CALM, COOL AND COLLECTED

On any routine day, after elective operations were finished, the residents gathered to view all the x-rays taken of patients in the intensive care unit (ICU). After that, we would make rounds, being sure to visit all of the patients. One particular day, the chief resident was sitting in front of the view box, surrounded by me and all the other residents. He grabbed a chest film of a patient who had an aortic coarctation [18] repaired by Dr. Gross that morning. When he put the x-ray in the view box, we were stunned—a little metallic bulldog clamp was left inside the patient's chest! The chief resident started crying like a child. Bulldog clamps were placed in the intercostal arteries and were supposed to be removed by the chief resident in charge of closing the patient's chest after Dr. Gross left the operating room. We did not know what to do. After exchanging several ideas, we all decided to go directly to Dr. Gross. We walked to his office and delivered the news.

We thought he would become agitated and scream but instead, a considerably cool Dr. Gross quietly instructed us to go back to the recovery room, take everyone by surprise and say that the patient was bleeding. Rush the patient into the operating room, open the chest, discreetly remove the clamp, "perform hemostasis"[19] and make the clamp disappear. We could not believe what Dr. Gross was suggesting but we firmly believed that he knew what he was doing. So, we walked into the recovery room, surrounded the patient and somebody yelled, "The patient is bleeding! Let's take him to the OR!" Everybody was mobilized.

The confused, perplexed, recovery room nurses simply followed our instructions. We hurried the patient into the operating room, put him to sleep, opened his chest and removed the bulldog clamp. The

18 A narrowing, compression or stricture of the walls of the body's main artery.

19 Procedure to control bleeding.

chief resident discretely dropped the clamp on the floor and put his foot on top of it. Then, a meticulous hemostasis was "performed," the chest was closed and the patient recovered uneventfully.

Afterwards, we were all in the surgeons' lounge recovering from our stressful incident. Suddenly, someone shouted, "What about the x-ray!" We looked at each other trying to come up with an answer. Again, we went back to Dr. Gross. "We did the job, Dr. Gross. The patient is doing very well. But what about the chest film?"

Dr. Gross simply said, "Get rid of it."

And who would be in charge of making the film disappear? One of the senior residents pointed out that there was only one person on our team who could leave the country in a hurry, if necessary. Everybody stared at me and I was "officially commissioned" to make the x-ray disappear. (And I did).

*****

First Ductus Ligation: Pioneered Operation Described by the Surgeon

For several years after Dr. Robert Gross retired, I would visit him in Vermont. He lived a very quiet life, giving me the impression that he was depressed. Whenever I would visit him for a couple of days he used to ask, "Alberto, did I ever tell you the story of the ductus arteriosus?"[20] And I always answered, "No, Dr. Gross. You never told me about that." Then, he would repeat a story that I enjoyed very much.

For those readers not familiar with the history of surgery, it is important to note that Dr. Robert E. Gross is perhaps the most prominent leader of pediatric surgery in the United States and perhaps the Western Hemisphere. He became a world celebrity because he was the first surgeon to successfully operate on a malformation that was considered incurable— the patent ductus arteriosus. (Ref. 4-6)

During his training, he spent an entire year in the pathology department[21] with Dr. S. Burt Wolbach, a prominent pathologist. Dr. Gross insisted that every surgical resident should spend time in the pathology department doing autopsies because that was a wonderful exercise for a future surgeon. This is where he saw a range of deceased patients that died from pulmonary hypertension[22] consecutive to a persistent patent ductus arteriosus. At that time, all patients with patent ductus arteriosus died because there was no treatment for that problem. There, in the autopsy room, is where Dr. Robert Gross conceived the idea of opening the chest and ligating[23] the ductus arteriosus. In the late 30s, opening the chest was extremely risky since the anesthesia was given by mask

---

20 Temporary fetal blood vessel that connects the aorta and the pulmonary artery.

21 Department in charge of the macro and microscopic study of tissues and post-mortem studies (autopsies).

22 Increased pressure in the arteries of the lung.

23 Procedure of tying off a blood vessel or duct with a suture or wire ligature.

without a tube passing through the trachea. Ventilation conducted with a mask represented a source of potential problems and complications. The operation had to be done skillfully and quickly and Dr. Gross believed that he could do it.

He went to Dr. William Ladd (his chief) and told him his plan. Dr. Ladd tried to dissuade him, "You are crazy! Don't try something like that. If you try and something goes wrong, you may lose your license. As a matter of fact, a pediatrician here recently lost his license because he attempted a new procedure on a baby and the baby died." The baby actually died from meningitis. The "new procedure" that was performed happened to be a spinal tap (lumbar puncture), commonly used today to diagnose meningitis.

Despite the warnings, Dr. Gross became increasingly obsessed with his idea. He discussed his plan with a prominent cardiologist named Paul D. White, who supported him. Then, Dr. Ladd went on vacation. Dr. Gross explained to me that he decided to book two cases for closure of the patent ductus arteriosus, one after the other, in two consecutive days. He thought that if he was at risk of losing his license, he deserved two chances. With the lessons he would learn from the first case, he would make the second one better. The first patient scheduled was a girl. Dr. Gross explained to the mother what he was going to do and the mother inquired, "How many cases have you done like this?"

Dr. Gross replied, "I hate to tell you, and if I do, you will never believe it. So, let's go ahead and do the operation."

On August 17th of 1938, Dr. Gross performed the operation and the patient survived! As a result, he decided to cancel the second scheduled case. At that point, his "series" included only one case but with a 100% survival rate. Why should he take a risk to decrease his results to 50% survival?

Days later, Dr. Gross went to a tennis game in Boston and by chance met Dr. Ladd, who was still on vacation. "Hi, Bob, what's going on at the hospital?"

"Many things are happening there, Sir. You will find out when you get back."

When Dr. Ladd returned from vacation, he found news about the new operation and the fact that the patient survived. From there, Dr. Gross rapidly became a world-famous surgeon. Perhaps that influenced the administration to appoint him Chief of Surgery when Dr. Ladd retired. This is a reason why surgeons like to say:

Do not argue with success.

Many years passed when I had the privilege to be invited back to Children's Hospital Boston to give the "Robert E. Gross Lecture." Sitting in the first row of the audience was a very proud lady who was the little girl that received the very first ligation of a patent ductus arteriosus by Dr. Gross.

BATHTUB EDUCATION

While on my visits in Vermont, Dr. Gross would also inquire, "Alberto, did I ever tell you the story of how I came up with the idea of repairing an atrioseptal defect?"

"No, Dr. Gross, you never told me about that."

Before Dr. John H. Gibbons, (Ref. 7) Dr. Walton Lillihei (Ref. 8) and others described the cardio-pulmonary bypass,[24] it was impossible to open the heart to repair an intracardiac defect. However, Dr. Gross used to repair atrioseptal defects[25] without cardio-pulmonary bypass. He knew that the venous pressure measured at the right atrium (central venous pressure or CVP)[26] was rather low; as a result, he conceived the idea to suture a waterproof well to the right atrium, allowing the blood from the right atrium to fill the well and, because the pressure in the right atrium is low, the blood stayed at a certain level within the well, without exsanguinating[27] the patient. At the same time, no air went into the heart or the coronary arteries. Then, Dr. Gross would put his hands into the blood of the well, palpate[28] the atrioseptal defect, ask for sutures and blindly patch the defect.

In Dr. Gross' home in Framingham, Massachusetts, they did not have showers. It was an old house where one could only have a bath while sitting in the tub. While bathing, the water becomes turbid and one cannot see through it. Many times he lost the soap in the water and had to find it using only the sensation of his fingers. He was amazed at how much he could "see" with his fingers, without

24 Procedure to divert the blood out of the body to oxygenate it and pump it back into the body.

25 Abnormal communication between the right and left atriums of the heart that allows the mixing of oxygenated and non-oxygenated blood.

26 Pressure of the blood in the veins and right atrium.

27 Extensive blood loss due to internal or external hemorrhage.

28 Part of physical exam in which an object is felt (usually with the hands) to determine its size, shape, firmness or location.

really seeing at all. That is where he got the idea for the repair of the atrioseptal defect!

The technique is magnificently illustrated in his classic book of pediatric surgery, *The Surgery of Infancy and Childhood.* (Ref. 1) The procedure became obsolete when the cardio-pulmonary bypass became available, which allowed safely opening the heart and repairing inner-heart defects more accurately. I remember that the head nurse of the ICU at Children's Boston, a young, healthy-looking lady, was one of those patients operated on by Dr. Gross when she was a child.

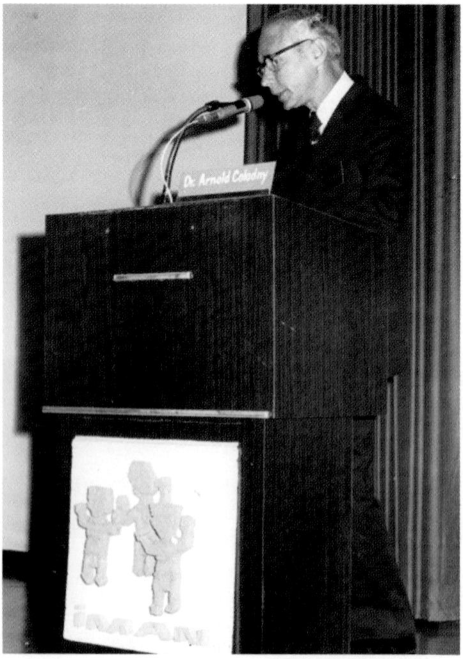

DR. ARNOLD COLODNY

When I was at Children's Boston, I met Dr. Arnold Colodny,

who was a member of the surgical staff. He struck me as a rather quiet, well-educated, respectful individual. I never heard about him prior to my arrival in the US. I must say now that he was the person from whom I learned the most during my training in Boston. Later in my life, having visited many children's hospitals in the US and abroad, I learned that it is common to find a surgeon who is famous because of his publications, his public appearances, his academic, administrative or political achievements. Frequently, in the same hospital, there is another surgeon who may not be as famous but is the one spending more time caring for patients, operating and teaching. One who has more moral authority in the actual practice of surgery and training residents. The person many would call when their own child needs an operation. I believe Dr. Colodny was such a person.

During conferences and meetings, every time he talked, I learned something. His figure kept growing and impressing me more and more each day. Even though my first impression of him was of a very serious person, later I could appreciate his great unique sense of humor. What I admired most about him was his mature, balanced judgment. When he spoke, we listened. He was not as famous as Dr. Gross but in my training he was more important. Dr. Colodny had a permanent ileostomy[29] and suffered from diabetes; yet, he worked as hard as any other member of the staff.

Plagued by many complicated and previously operated cases,

29 Diversion of stool through an orifice in the abdominal wall into a plastic bag.

referred to him because of his excellent reputation, Dr. Colodny used to say, humorously:

If you are going to do an operation that is not indicated, you better do it right.

It may be difficult to believe but some patients are subjected to unnecessary operations that are not indicated and they are not done properly.

I remember one particular event that portrays Dr. Colodny's personality quite well. I was assisting him with a complex case and after many hours of working with the patient's unusually complicated anatomy, I heard Dr. Colodny say, "What do you suggest to do?"

I looked behind me and around me, trying to find whom he was talking. To my surprise, he was actually asking me! In those years, particularly at the Central Military Hospital in Mexico, professors rarely asked the residents what should be done. Residents assumed their opinions were not relevant and that the professors knew everything. When I realized that the question was directed to me, I was forced to think more carefully about what was occurring in the operative field.[30] All at once, I was no longer a simple spectator assisting a surgeon. He made me part of the team. Then, in my own brain, I began to visualize and conceive technical alternatives that could be useful in the case and finally expressed my opinion. I remember that as a great illuminating event. This is something that

30 The area that is open during surgery.

surgeons should try to repeat during operations when assisted by a trainee. It makes the resident feel important and it forces him to use his intellect and concentrate on what is happening in the operative field: the essential components of good surgical training.

*****

Dr. Colodny invited my family to stay at his home while he attended a pediatric surgical meeting in the Bahamas and care for his dog, Brutus (the largest English mastiff that I have ever seen). It was with great reservations that I went there with three frightened little children but Brutus turned out to be a lovely, beautiful animal. Dr. Colodny and his wife were expected to spend a week in the Bahamas but, unfortunately, they came back much earlier because he had an accident while riding a motorcycle and seriously injured his knee. They flew back on an emergency basis and he was operated on at Peter Bent Brigham Hospital. Even though the operation was successful, he was told not to stand on that knee for several months. That was devastating news for him because he needed to continue operating due to financial concerns.

Dr. Colodny then meticulously planned to continue his operations without stepping on that particular foot. His wife made special scrubs for him—they were fashioned with a zipper in the lateral part of the pants so he could change his clothes in the locker room while on crutches, without assistance. Dr. Colodny also choreographed a series of very ingenious maneuvers to be able to work in the operating room. Using several weekends, he went alone to the locker room to practice changing his clothes and scrubbing while on crutches, putting weight on only one foot. I tried to help him but he refused; he wanted to do it himself.

Finally, without assistance and on one foot, Dr. Colodny learned to change his clothes and wear scrubs. He used the crutches to walk from the locker room to the OR. There, he scrubbed while standing on the healthy foot; the crutches were placed against the wall. Next, the scrub nurse came and dressed him with the sterile gown and gloves while he was still on one foot. He grabbed the crutches with his sterile gloves and hobbled to the operating room. Inside the OR, the scrub nurse removed the contaminated gown and gloves and redressed him using new sterile garments. Then, he started the operation standing on one foot. If he got tired, he would sit on a high stool for a few minutes and continue the operation. This went on for several months and his mood was always the same: calm and confident.

Dr. Colodny was an admirable person, to say the least. He represented the kind of professor that everybody should have—someone to be able to call in the middle of the night because there is a problem with a patient. Under those circumstances, a highly respected individual, offering a balanced, honest opinion is needed. When I went back to Mexico, I called Dr. Colodny many times because I knew that he was that kind of person.

TACOS

I invited Dr. Colodny to Mexico to give lectures. On this particular occasion he traveled with his entire family. Dining out, I tried to take them to good restaurants because I was particularly concerned with Dr. Colodny's medical problems and I did not want him or his family to suffer a "tourist disease." Many tourists who ate Mexican food in unclean places were afflicted with severe diarrhea and dehydration also known as "Montezuma's revenge." A person with an ileostomy would be at a much higher risk for a more severe case.

Sure enough, from day one, Dr. Colodny had a taste for Mexico, "Alberto, I want to go to a real *taquería* (restaurant specializing in tacos) and try authentic tacos." I pretended that I did not hear him well and changed the subject. However, every morning, Dr. Colodny made the same request. So, I devised a plan.

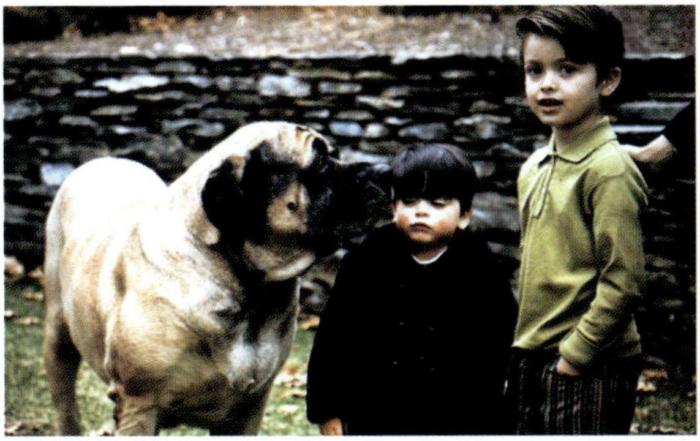

Brutus making friends with my children

I estimated the incubation period of the bacteria that produces

"Montezuma's revenge" to be around six hours—a little more time than the flight to Boston. I waited until the day of their departure while we were on our way to the airport to fulfill the doctor's wish. I figured that if Dr. Colodny got sick, he would be safer in Boston. Dr. Colodny was lucky though; he ate many tacos at lunch and did not experience "Montezuma's revenge." He loved the tacos.

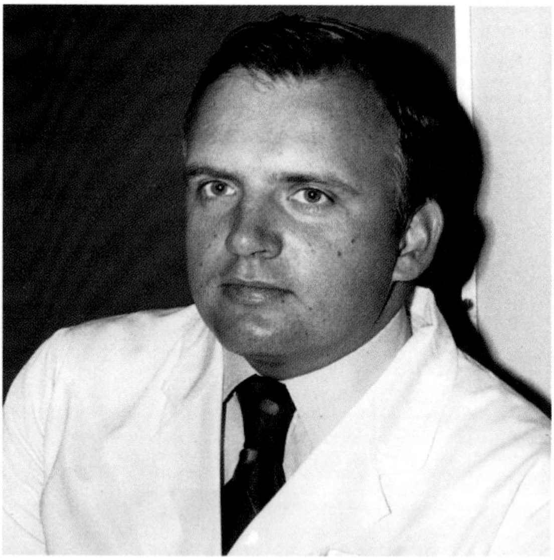

DR. WILLIS WILLIAMS

Dr. Willis Williams and I worked together as fellows at Children's Hospital Boston. He came from Massachusetts General Hospital (Mass General). Even when we both were pediatric surgical fellows, he was the official one, because of the circumstances in which I became a fellow. He was also my chief, even though Willis is one or two years younger than me. I found Willis to be a marvelous person (he is still one of my best friends). I admire him because of his professional talent, his sensitivity and his moral integrity. Willis Williams decided to adopt me as a trainee. He protected me. He was patient and tolerant with my errors. He trusted me and made me feel secure.

I remember one day, I saw a baby in the emergency room with an incarcerated hernia.[31] I manually reduced the hernia and decided to admit the baby to operate on him the next day. I called the admitting office to make the necessary arrangements, only to find that the lady who answered the phone claimed, for various bureaucratic reasons, that there was no way for me to do so. I insisted that it was very important to admit the baby at that particular time. We had a heated discussion and then I heard her cover the phone, "I am talking to one of those foreign guys and he's giving me trouble."

While I was talking to her, Dr. Williams was in front of me. Obviously, my face changed because when I hung up he asked what was wrong. I explained it to him and he was very upset, but he did not say a word. He disappeared. About 10 minutes later, he came back. "The lady you were talking to on the phone is going to come to see you and apologize."

"Willis, you did not have to do that."

Two minutes later, the same lady phoned me, "Dr. Peña, where are you? I want to talk to you and apologize."

"I accept your apology. You do not have to come here."

But she insisted. She came and happened to be a very nice

31 Condition in which an organ or body part, such as the intestine, protrudes through an opening in the body structure that normally contains and cannot be easily reduced.

person; she started crying in front of me. "I apologize for what I said about you being a foreign guy. Dr. Williams came to my office and asked for my name. My name is of German origin and he reminded me that most of us in this country were foreigners at some point, because this is a country of immigrants. Dr. Williams also reminded me, immigrant or not, you are a senior resident of this hospital trying to help a baby. He asked me to apologize and that is what I am doing. I sincerely hope you will forgive me." She was still crying. I was moved and felt really embarrassed. I did not know what to do so I said some words, trying to make her feel better.

*****

On a weekend day that I was on-call, Willis walked into the hospital and found me. "Alberto, go home, have lunch with your family and come back in the evening, I'll cover for you."

"Why, Willis? I am here doing all right. I'm happy."

"This is an order."

So, I went home to rest and spend time with my family.

In addition to being a great surgeon and obsessive worker, Dr. Willis Williams was an extraordinary photographer, an excellent piano player, a sensitive, humane and above all, excellent friend. We continued our friendship and I had the pleasure of inviting him to Mexico so that my residents could meet him. He became a pediatric cardiac surgeon and then he invited me to Eggleston Children's Hospital in Atlanta when he was chief of surgery there. I will always be grateful to Dr. Willis Williams for what I have learned from him, because of his exemplary professionalism and the privilege of his friendship.

Willis Williams was very much influenced by Hardy Hendren of Mass General. His camera was exactly like the one Hardy used, as well as his surgical instruments. Because of Willis' influence on me, before I went back to Mexico, I wanted to buy the same type of camera and same set of surgical instruments (including a bronchoscope, cystoscope and esophagoscope)—all indispensible tools that any good pediatric surgeon should have. I knew it would be difficult to obtain these instruments in Mexico.

To purchase these tools, Victor Scalise advised me to go to my local bank to ask for a loan. The bankers, he suggested, would be very happy to lend money to a young surgeon trained at Children's Boston. So, I went to the bank.

The bank director welcomed me into his office and I introduced myself as Dr. Peña. I explained to him that I would be finishing my training very soon and I needed money to purchase some medical equipment.

"Let me assure you, Dr. Peña. You are in the right place."

Our conversation went on for several minutes and he expressed his admiration for the kind of work we were doing at Children's Boston. He asked how much money I required and I told him I needed $12,000.

"Not a problem, Dr. Peña." And the director called an assistant to prepare the loan. "I wish you all the best with your professional future. And just out of curiosity, where will you be practicing?"

"In Mexico," I replied.

"New Mexico, huh?"

"No, I said Mexico."

At this point his face changed. "Mexico? Oh no, I am sorry, Dr. Peña. The bank is unable to lend money to someone who is living abroad."

But, like Alexander Graham Bell said:

When one door closes, another opens.

The money I needed did not come from any bank. It came as a loan from Dr. Carrillo, a doctor who practiced in the mountains of the Mexican state of Puebla. He and my brother-in-law, Dr. Alfonso Velasco, used to invite me to assist them in operations when I was a medical student. I will be forever indebted to the both of them for their generosity.

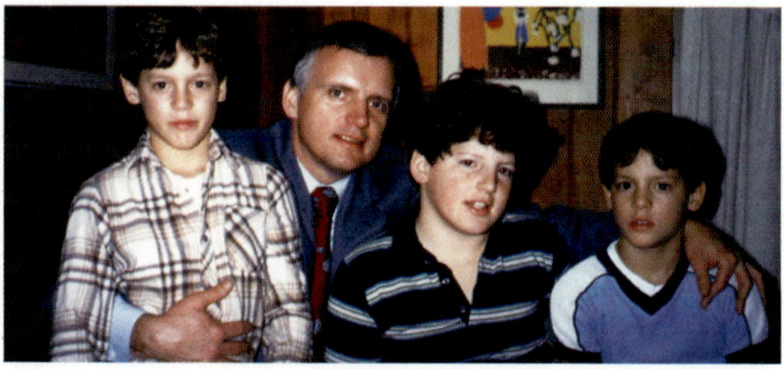

Willis Williams and his children: Robert, Eric, and Christopher

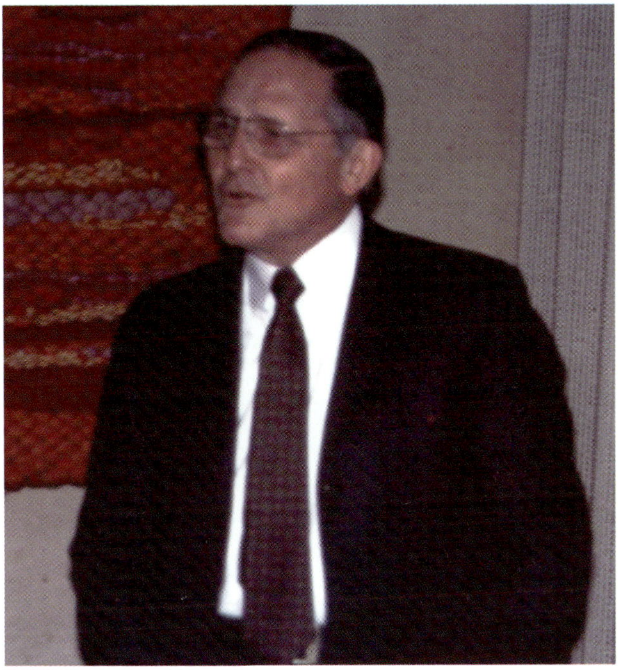

DR. HARDY HENDREN

Another influential figure in my career was Dr. Hardy Hendren, a very famous pediatric surgeon. When I was at Children's Hospital Boston, I would frequently hear the name Hardy Hendren—the surgeons at the hospital whispered about him. Hardy Hendren received his training under Dr. Gross at Children's Hospital Boston. When he finished his training, he stayed there as an attending surgeon. Eventually, Dr. Gross fired him. Most people agreed that Dr. Hendren was fired because he was becoming "too busy," which apparently made Dr. Gross feel insecure. Dr. Hendren went on to Massachusetts General Hospital, just minutes away from "the Mecca" of pediatric surgery (Children's Hospital Boston), established his own practice and developed a reputation of being technically better than most surgeons in the area, including those from Children's.

When I met Dr. Willis Williams, he said, "Alberto, I want you to call Dr. Hardy Hendren's secretary, use my name. Tell her that I have sent you to observe Dr. Hendren in the OR and you can only do it in the evenings because of your work. Ask her to give you the dates and types of operations that Dr. Hendren is doing."

Being fellows at Children's Hospital we were not supposed to go to Mass General (or any other hospital) to learn pediatric surgery but Willis Williams considered it imperative for me and I did exactly that, but discreetly. Hardy Hendren worked very long hours every day; thus, it was easy for a fellow on his day off to take a taxi to watch him. He welcomed me and I learned many things. I was never officially his fellow or resident but, from a technical standpoint, he is one of the surgeons who influenced me the most.

Hardy Hendren taught me that surgeons must fight for what they believe; they must be persistent in order to repair a malformation. Surgeons should not leave the operating room until they are happy and comfortable with the operation. Even if a surgeon has been working many hours, if not satisfied, they have to take down every single stitch and redo the whole operation again, until content. I have never met another person who was so obsessive and meticulous. Hardy was rather intimidating but one of the best technical surgeons that I have ever seen. He is the type of surgeon that loves to operate. Years after, I invited him to Mexico several times to repair complex malformations and it was always an eye-opening scene.

THE HARDY WAY

There are so many anecdotes related to Hardy Hendren that in any pediatric surgical meeting or reunion, if one wanted to create a subject of conversation, just mentioning the name Hardy Hendren would do it.

When I was back in Mexico, I took some private patients requiring complex operations to Mass General to be operated on by Hardy Hendren. On one of those occasions, I called Hardy the night before to find out where we should meet. "I'll wait for you at 6:30 a.m. at the entrance of Mass General."

I was there at 6:30 sharp. Hardy was already there, holding a briefcase full of pens with writing on them that read, "Hardy Hendren says, 'Smoking will kill you.'"

We started jogging from the entrance of Mass General to his office. On the way, we saw a man who was smoking. Hardy stopped, snatched the cigarette away from the man's mouth and threw it on the ground. He opened his briefcase and gave him a pen, closed the briefcase and continued jogging toward his office.

*****

During one of his visits to Mexico, Hardy Hendren was giving a lecture to the Mexican Association of Urologists. Before he started, he unbuttoned his shirt and showed everybody a scar that he had on his abdomen, "Look! You see this! I got this scar, gentlemen, because I had cancer. I used to smoke. After I had this operation, I promised that I would fight against smoking."

At that point, all the surgeons who were smoking got the hint and started putting out their cigarettes. Once everyone stopped, Hardy started his lecture. Like most gatherings, there is always someone who is tardy and that night was no exception. A urologist arrived late and lighted a cigarette. Hardy noticed the smoke filtering through the light of the projector and stopped his speech. "Lights, please! Lights!"

He screamed at the surgeon, "You! I am talking to you," pointing with his finger toward the now pale, intimidated urologist. "Stop smoking! Didn't you hear what I said before?" The poor late coming urologist shrank, put his cigarette out and disappeared.

*****

When I was in Long Island, NY, I invited Hardy to be a guest speaker during one of the courses on anorectal malformations that I organized every 6 months. Pediatric surgeons from all over the world attended the course. That particular time, there was a Russian pediatric surgeon in the audience. During one of the coffee breaks, the Russian surgeon approached Hardy to ask him a technical question and in his pocket he carried a package of cigarettes that anyone could see. Before he said a word, Hardy grabbed the package from his shirt pocket, squeezed them in his powerful hand and threw it in the garbage can. "This is the first day of your new life, free of smoking."

I was afraid of the Russian surgeon's reaction but he did not say a word and did not ask the question that he (and everyone else) had in mind. Often, I was concerned that somebody would be angry with Hardy but he did all those things in such a self-confident way, taking people by surprise, that usually nobody said a word to him.

AN HONEST CONSIDERATION

When I came up with the idea of approaching patients with anorectal malformations in a different way, one of the first things that I decided to do was to go to Boston and show Hardy. He was an obsessive, perfectionist technician. I felt that he would be the person who would appreciate my idea the most and also give me a valuable criticism about my proposal. I put together all my slides plus my nonprofessional, super 8 movie films and flew from Mexico City to visit him at Mass General. Hardy was an extremely busy person. I thought that perhaps he would not have time to listen to me, watch my movies and see my slides.

Despite of all his responsibilities, he and I went to a room alone, "Alright, Alberto, show me what you have." And so, for two uninterrupted hours, he watched everything and listened intently, urging me to show him more. When I finished my presentation, he offered, "Alberto, this approach is going to be the preferred approach for the treatment of anorectal malformations in about eight years."

"Why eight years, Hardy? Why not now?"

"Because it takes about eight years to introduce a new technique. Surgeons don't like to change. It's going to take eight years, provided you use good audiovisual material and not this garbage that you have." So, I went back to Mexico and worked hard to have better audiovisual material, particularly because I was working in an anatomic area that was not known by most surgeons.

*****

Eventually, Hardy Hendren and I were, in a way, competing with each other because we worked in the surgical treatment of female patients born with cloacae.[32] Hardy made a tremendous contribution to the management of this complex malformation. (Ref. 9) It was always an honor for me to hear Hardy Hendren discussing my papers in pediatric surgical meetings. When I presented the new approach and technique for the first time in the *American Pediatric Surgical Association* meeting, Hardy approached me a few minutes before and offered some advice, "There are some people in the audience who are going to make very negative, nasty

32 Malformations occurring in females with a common cavity in which the intestinal, genital and urinary tracts open. See page 121 for further discussion of cloacae.

comments about your presentation. Don't be upset. Don't be angry and don't argue with them. You just say, 'I just presented, for your consideration, another way to treat these patients.''' Sure enough, there was an angry looking surgeon who made a negative comment about my presentation. I answered only what Hardy had advised me to answer.

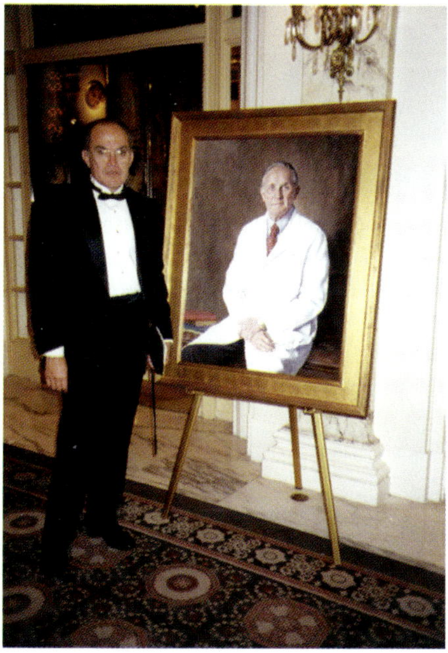

Dr. Peña at the occasion of Dr. Hendren's retirement

I will always be in debt to Hardy Hendren for his teaching. In addition, when I was invited to become chief of pediatric surgery at Schneider Children's Hospital Long Island Jewish Medical Center in New York, the Board of Regents for the New York State Education Department requested letters of recommendation to grant me a license to practice within the state. I gave the name of several

American surgeons, including Hardy Hendren. The best letter of recommendation came from Hardy Hendren. I feel an enormous gratitude towards this brilliant surgeon.

*****

Adding to all of the talented, inspiring personalities influencing me throughout my life, I feel very much in debt with many individuals who go unnamed. Some surgeons do not like to publish papers. They do not talk much. They do not occupy leadership positions. They are not famous. Yet, these excellent surgeons and magnificent human beings are determined to work hard for their specialty. I am eternally grateful for the hospitality and confidence shown to me when invited to their countries to operate on the most treasured members of their society: their children.

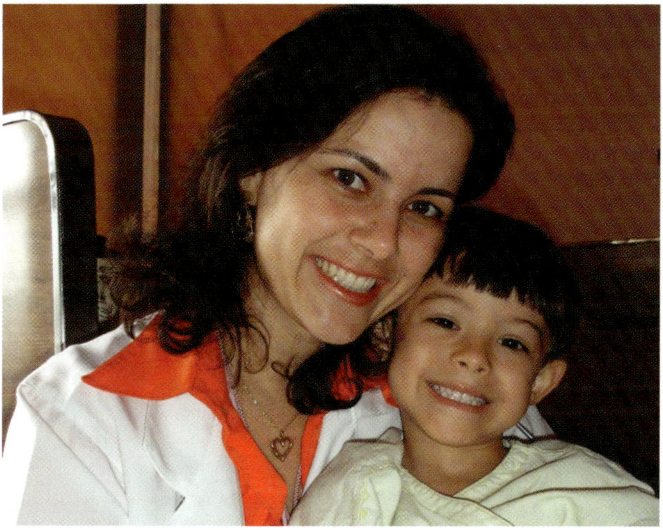

Dr. Andrea Bischoff and patient

BITTEN BY THE SPIDER

Throughout life, there are certain events that alter an individual's entire perspective about the world. I remember reading the biography of a famous American musician. He described a time when he was a child, playing baseball in his neighborhood. When he was holding the bat, ready to hit the ball, he suddenly heard a beautiful melody coming from somewhere. He dropped the bat and walked, hypnotized, toward the sound. He remained near the house where the music was playing and could not move until the melody had finished. Up to that moment, that extremely sensitive and talented boy had no formal musical education but he was so greatly touched by the event that his life transformed on that day. Eventually, he became a world-renowned musician and composer.

The same thing may happen to anybody while contemplating a painting that produces tremendous emotion, shaking the soul or while reading a book with revealing new ideas and descriptions that touch the inner most feelings. It may occur while pondering philosophical concepts that are fulfilling and fascinating or when meeting an extraordinary human being. Any of these chance encounters may completely influence a person's path in life.

As I mentioned before, in 1965, I went to Children's Hospital Boston with my son, Gustavo, who had biliary atresia. There, I had my first opportunity to observe Dr. Gross operate. Before that moment, I was mostly exposed to adult general surgical procedures with very little exposure to pediatric operations. As most surgeons know, there is an enormous discrepancy between techniques, approaches, handling of tissues, development of planes, instruments, blood loss and the trauma inflicted on an adult patient and pediatric patient. I already knew that I loved children but I was still uncertain about my professional future.

I remember watching Dr. Gross perform an open-heart operation. The operation progressed silently; very few words were exchanged during the entire procedure. I was deeply impressed by the precision of his movements, how smooth the entire procedure was and how the scrub nurse anticipated every single movement of the operation, handing Dr. Gross the right instrument at the right time. To me, this played out like a concert performed by a symphony orchestra. I was "bitten by the spider," never to recover.

To better understand the impact of that event in my career, keep in mind that my previous experience had mainly been with adult general surgical procedures; some of them performed by efficient and effective surgeons and many others conducted by very rough surgeons. Watching the harsh operations was not very easy for me; I could not understand what those surgeons were trying to do. I thought that surgery was very complicated because I saw surgeons sweating, screaming, cursing and blaming the scrub nurse, the assistant or the anesthesiologist[33] for everything that went awry. I even remember a professor of mine in desperation, in the middle of a "difficult" operation, stop, open his arms and look to the ceiling, "Oh God, please send me a good assistant. Take away this donkey that is trying to assist me."

After my first, brief time at Children's Boston, I returned to Mexico to finish my training but I could not recover from that experience. That rather romantic event turned out to influence my professional life and have much more relevance than I first thought. I decided then that I wanted to be a pediatric surgeon. I promised myself that I would not only be a good pediatric surgeon but I would strive to be one who will always try to imitate the beautiful concert-like procedure I had seen. This induced me to seek further training in Boston in 1969.

33 A medical specialist who administers an agent (anesthetic) that reversibly depresses neuronal function, producing total or partial loss of sensation to a patient before being treated.

Later in my life I was lucky enough to become a professor of pediatric surgery and to be invited to perform operations in many places all over the world. Many young surgeons and medical students have observed my operations and I like to believe that I have influenced their professional lives just as I was with Dr. Gross and his ensemble.

It is extremely flattering to receive a letter from a surgeon relating that watching or assisting in an operation, significantly changed the perspective of his career. This is a serious responsibility, particularly because during many operations, there is always somebody—medical student, resident or visitor—watching. This is very important to keep in mind for all surgeons. In the OR of most hospitals, there is a silent medical student or intern who knows little about surgery; he can become fascinated and inspired by a good operation or despondent and horrified by a surgical field that looks like an explosion in a meat factory. Surgeons must be very careful with their behavior—watching every comment and checking attitudes at the door. The young people watching learn not only the good things but also the bad. Negative, rough, careless surgeons should not practice in the presence of young individuals. Pessimistic, as well as cynical comments, must be avoided during an operation, particularly in an academic environment.

*****

I remember giving a lecture in a South American country. A doctor who had just finished medical school six months before, came to me after the presentation and asked many intelligent questions while walking with me to my hotel. He then inquired if I was going to operate in his country. "Yes, as a matter of fact, tonight at 9 p.m. I will not be attending the banquet because I was invited to operate on a patient in a government hospital." He asked if he could attend and I answered, "Of course, as far as I am concerned, you can be there. I do not know what kind of requirements the hospital has for young doctors from other institutions to enter the operating room." Surprisingly, that night, when I entered the operating room, the young man was already scrubbed. He had managed to make the necessary arrangements to not only watch but to scrub in as a second assistant.

The surgeon assigned to assist me that night was a fully trained pediatric surgeon but was not particularly familiar with the technique to repair the malformation. Although the young visiting doctor was not trained in surgery, within a few minutes of the operation, he understood the basic steps and general strategy of the procedure. Gradually, he intruded more and more into the territory of the first assistant, pushing him away from the surgical field. With no previous training, this young man turned out to be an excellent surgical assistant.

We finished the operation around midnight and he asked what I was doing the next morning. I told him that I was invited to another city to operate on three major cases. Therefore, I was going to rest and very early the next morning, I would board a plane because the city was about 450 miles away. Again, he asked if he could attend the operations and I said, as far as I was concerned, he could. From that hospital, sometime after midnight, the young doctor went to the bus terminal and took an overnight charter to arrive early in the morning in the other city.

When I entered the operating room, he was there! In spite of his highly confident attitude and persistence, he was not allowed to scrub in but he did spend the entire day watching over my shoulder, observing all three of the operations. When I finished, the local surgeons offered me a party and I invited the young doctor. But he said he had to take a bus that night to go back home. I never heard from him again. I hope he is doing a good job operating on many patients somewhere in South America. Similar things have happened to me all over the world. It is tremendously satisfying to know that in my professional life I was able to replicate in others, the experience that I had while watching Dr. Gross in 1965.

THE STORY OF THE POSTERIOR SAGITTAL APPROACH

In 1980, I conceived a new way to approach the surgical repair of anorectal malformations in children—a surgical procedure to create a functional anus and rectum by approaching the area through a midline incision made in between both buttocks. This technique is now well-known among pediatric surgeons all over the world as posterior sagittal anorectoplasty (PSARP) or Peña procedure. Since that time, I gradually became more involved in the surgical treatment of various anorectal malformations and colorectal problems in children. Because of my contribution I have had the privilege of traveling, giving lectures and operating in many countries. Very often, in almost every place I go, there is a young surgeon eager to hear the story of how I came up with the idea for the new approach.

Whenever the famous Argentinean writer Jose Luis Borges was

asked to write his autobiography, he refused, insisting that human beings always fabricate or invent their own story, modifying the truth to make it more liked, consciously or subconsciously, deleting episodes that are not favorable. Being human, I do not expect to be an exception.

When another famous writer, Nobel Prize winner Pablo Neruda, was specifically asked about this subject he answered, "It is not that I lie, I just make little changes to the truth to make it better." I guess the same may happen here.

LEARNING CURVES

Of course, I have thought a lot about this and I believe the story actually began when I was a medical student. During the following years, I was exposed to many interesting experiences leaving me with a healthy skepticism that, when combined with my natural curiosity and imagination, determined how the idea originated.

Imagination is more important than knowledge. ~Albert Einstein

At the Military Medical School in Mexico, students had to work hard; otherwise, they would be dismissed from the school (a serious defeat) only to attend another medical school and possibly receive lower quality training. Some students, without enough resources, had to work a part-time job to support themselves and pay for schooling. As a consequence, everyone studied in a rather obsessive way.

The Military Medical School was a great school. Thinking

back though, if I could make a suggestion to improve the measure of teaching at my Alma Mater, it would be for the professors to display a more encouraging and positive attitude towards the students. In those years, students basically learned to repeat what the professors said. We were not encouraged to question what we read or what was said. Nor were we encouraged to have an independent judgment. We were not stimulated to analyze what we learned. Creativity was not encouraged or inspired. We were not instructed to be skeptical about the books we read, to look into the original sources, to scrutinize the articles of literature that were quoted, critically analyzing the sources of the statements. This was particularly true when the textbooks were written in English. Every student was simply searching for strategies and techniques to pass and stay in school, not so much to comprehend or understand. The struggle was to memorize and repeat during the examinations what the book and the professor said in class.

Growing up in a so-called "underdeveloped" or "developing country" brings additional disadvantages to medical students and young doctors. A major disadvantage is sometimes reflected in the manner professors teach the students. Living in Mexico, most of the medical literature came from the United States. In developing countries, there is a tendency for the doctors to be polarized. In one extreme are the ultranationalist xenophobes who are opposed to everything that comes from other countries. In the opposite extreme are doctors who only believe in what comes from developed countries and have a basic primary mistrust of anything created in their own country. New generations of students, not only in medicine but also in every discipline, should be instructed to search for the truth, regardless of its origin. They should be taught that science, as well as art, has no frontiers, nationalities or ideologies.

Like in most medical schools, there were some excellent professors, others were mediocre and some were definitely very bad. Some professors tried to explain things and did it so awkwardly that I actually could not understand a word they said. My classmates made fun of me because many times, after the professor gave an explanation, I raised my hand and argued or said that I could not understand. By doing that, I extended the length of the class and frequently exasperated my classmates. My memory was never very good and it was always a struggle for me to memorize things that I could not understand. Some of my classmates had excellent memories, which made me feel uncomfortable and I really underestimated my intellectual capacity. I felt that I was limited because I could not grasp many things that my classmates seemed to understand so well. In retrospect, I like to repeat a popular truth:

It is preferable to endure a minute of embarrassment
rather than a whole life of ignorance.

After I finished medical school, I became an intern at the Central Military Hospital. During my rotation in the department of pulmonology and thoracic surgery (non-cardiac),[34] I was involved in lobar resections[35] and reducing thoracoplasties[36] in patients suffering from tuberculosis.[37] It was the intern's responsibility to write all of the operative reports by hand. On one of my first days in that department, after one of these operations, I recorded that a "Veork thoracoplasty" was performed. My senior resident reviewed my note and mocked me, saying that I did not write it correctly and that it actually was a "Viorc thoracoplasty." The next day, the chief resident participated in the controversy and declared that the correct way to write it was "Beorc thoracoplasty." The discussion came up during patients' rounds, so we asked the attending surgeons and each one of them came up with a different spelling for the name of the surgeon who described the thoracoplasty. I volunteered myself to research the original paper.

Back then it was not easy to locate an original source. There were no computers. I went to the hospital library but could not find the paper. Somebody suggested that I visit the Instituto de Neumología (Pulmonology Institute) in Mexico City to search. One night I went there and found the original paper in a Scandinavian Journal. I was surprised to find that all of us were wrong, including the chief of the department! That operation was performed everyday, but nobody

---

34 Branches of medicine, respectively, that deal with diseases of the respiratory system and diseases and injuries of the thoracic area, including the lungs and respiratory tract.

35 Removal of part of the lung.

36 Techniques to reduce the size of the chest to be adapted to the smaller volume of the lung.

37 Potentially fatal contagious disease that can affect almost any part of the body but is mainly an infection of the lungs

was writing it correctly. The surgeon's name was Björk; thus, the procedure is known as Björk's thoracoplasty. (Ref. 10) That day I discovered that a little bit of healthy skepticism could be very useful in the practice of medicine.

*****

A second episode occurred during a long thoracic operation of a lobectomy[38] on a soldier. As an intern, I was the second assistant. The second assistant could see very little of what was happening in the operative field because they were expected to hold a retractor[39] for several long, tedious hours. In order to avoid being too bored while holding the retractor, I recommend pondering an interesting subject for that time, doing nothing.

My gaze was locked, staring at the x-ray of the soldier's chest, trying to visualize the patient's position on the table. To my recollection, the patient was on his right side and we were opening the left side of his chest. The x-ray showed that the lesion on the lung was in the right side. We were opening the wrong side! It was with great hesitation that I decided to interrupt the colonel professor and his first assistant, "I am sorry, Sir, but I am afraid that we're opening the wrong side of the chest."

The professor scoffed, "Are you trying to be funny? Keep the

---

38 In this case, an operation on the chest for the excision of one part of the lung.

39 Instrument for holding back the edges of tissues and organs to maintain exposure of the underlying anatomic parts.

retractor steady and keep your mouth shut."

So, that is exactly what I did. However, I could not stop contemplating the problem. The more I thought, the more sure I was that we were on the wrong side. After about 10 or 15 minutes, already inside the chest, I interjected again, "I am sorry but I think this is the wrong side."

The surgeon finally stopped, looked at the film, compared it with the patient's position and agreed with me. He started cursing. The patient eventually came out of the operating room with double incisions in his chest! That day, I learned that professors may be wrong and surgery is unforgiving when surgeons do not pay complete attention to the details.

*****

When I was a junior resident at Children's Hospital Boston, I was assigned to assist a very prominent pediatric surgeon in a cystoscopy.[40] Routinely, the surgeon allowed the resident to pass the cystoscope[41] and describe what he saw. In those days, only the person who held the cystoscope could see through the instrument. There were no TV screens connected to the device. The professor allowed me to see first, "Describe what you see."

I tried to see but everything was dark. I manipulated the

40 Procedure in which a delicate optical instrument (cystoscope) is passed through the urethra for diagnostic purposes.

41 A tubular instrument equipped with a light used to examine the interior of the urinary bladder and ureter.

instrument, checked the light, checked everything and looked again. It was still dark. The surgeon was growing impatient, "What do you see?"

"Sir, I only see darkness."

Nearly exasperated, he finally took over, "Take a pen. I'll dictate what I find." He went on to describe a normal urethra,[42] the characteristics of the bladder neck,[43] the trigone[44] and the ureteral orifices.[45] He removed the device, removed his gloves, gave me a few post-operative instructions and triumphantly walked out of the operating room. I felt humiliated and very upset. I took the scope again and tried to look through it but it was still dark. I disassembled the scope and was very surprised to find that someone put a very short 30°-angle telescope into the very long cystoscope sheath; therefore, it was impossible to view anything. Here I was, coming from Mexico where things were less than perfect, only to find that things like this happen in the US as well! I was learning to be skeptical and to believe in my own perceptions.

*****

In 1974, while I was chief of surgery at INP (now known as National Institute of Pediatrics), I read a paper by a prominent

42 Canal that carries urine from the bladder to the outside of the body. In the male it also serves as a genital duct.

43 Constricted portion of the urinary bladder that contributes to avoid leakage of urine.

44 Triangular region of the wall of the urinary bladder, the three angles corresponding with the orifices of the ureters and urethra.

45 Openings of uterers into the urinary bladder at the corners of the trigone of the bladder..

American surgeon about an experimental study done with rabbits. In the study, one group of rabbits, artificially depleted of platelets,[46] received an injection of endotoxin[47] while another similar group of rabbits, with normal platelets, received the same amount of endotoxin. The rate of death (mortality) in the rabbits without platelets was significantly higher than in those with normal platelet counts. The study included the level of endotoxins in the animals' blood measured with a limulus test in which the hemolymph[48] of the limulus crab (horseshoe crab) was mixed with the serum of the patient. Any presence of endotoxins provoked turbidity and its magnitude reflected the level of endotoxins. The study suggested that platelets, in addition to their role in coagulation, probably had another protective function in sequestrating the endotoxin and transporting it to the reticuloendothelial system[49] to be destroyed. In other words, the platelets could play a very significant role in the treatment of endotoxemias.[50]

At INP there were a large number of septic pediatric patients who died from sepsis,[51] either from severe diarrhea and/or perforation of the small bowel or the colon. It was assumed that these patients suffered from severe endotoxemia and frequently they had low platelet counts. The study suggested, that by measuring the level of

---

46 Cells in the blood with an important role in coagulation.

47 Potentially toxic natural compounds found inside pathogens, such as bacteria.

48 Bloodlike fluid of invertebrates having open blood-vascular systems.

49 Part of the immune system that pertains to the lymph nodes.

50 Presence of potentially toxic natural compounds in the blood.

51 Severe infection caused by pathogenic organisms, especially bacteria, in the blood or tissues.

endotoxin with the limulus test and infusing platelets, the patients could improve their bodies' response to the endotoxemia.

I decided to call the author of the paper in the United States and have a conversation with him. I explained that INP had many poor patients with sepsis and most likely severe endotoxemia. If he was interested in repeating his experiences in humans, we could measure the amount of endotoxin in our patients and consider injecting platelets before and after the measurement of the level of endotoxins. For that, it would be necessary to send one of the members of his research team (a Ph.D. and co-author of the paper) and all the necessary equipment to perform the limulus tests to Mexico.

It was an ambitious project; it was also difficult considering the restrictions that customs imposed in Mexico. I talked to the director, who had a direct connection with the president of Mexico's wife, and we were granted permission to introduce the laboratory equipment from the United States for a one-month study at INP. I also managed to secure a room in the laboratory of the hospital that would be used just for the Ph.D. to conduct the tests. We designed a protocol that consisted in obtaining blood from septic patients and sending it to the visitor's laboratory for him to measure the level of endotoxin. We also measured the number of platelets. At the end of one month, we were supposed to correlate the clinical evolution of the patients with the level of endotoxin and the number of platelets. With high hopes, perhaps the second stage of the project could consider the administration of platelets in very sick patients. We were very excited.

The scientist arrived. I personally welcomed him at the airport to be sure that there were no bureaucratic obstacles. He started working right away. My surgical residents were alerted about our protocol and were instructed to send blood samples of very sick patients. I was curious to see how the limulus test was done. Every morning I managed to spend a few minutes watching the scientist work, asking him many questions. It was not easy for me to understand but the whole test seemed to be extremely subjective, which awakened my skepticism. I had an idea: I had some of my very loyal surgical residents secretly donate their blood and send it to the laboratory under the names of our patients. For a month, we were secretly alternating samples of blood of very sick patients with samples of very healthy surgical residents.

By the end of the study, the researcher was very pleased with the results: the levels of endotoxin were very high in all samples! He said that he would do the statistical analysis and there would most likely be a good publication. He was ready to return to the United States. I invited him to a farewell dinner. During the dinner I told him the truth about the study. He got extremely upset. He left Mexico and I never heard from him. I made a special trip to United States to talk to his chief and explain what happened. Nothing more was ever heard about the limulus test in septic patients with low platelet counts. Again, I was learning to be skeptical and question everything that I read and heard.

BLIND BELIEVERS

When I was a research fellow at Children's Boston, a new clinical surgical fellow arrived from Melbourne, Australia. His name was Dr. Justin Kelly. He was already a trained pediatric surgeon in Australia; yet, he wanted to continue his training for two more years at Children's Boston. I worked closely with him and we became good friends. Dr. Kelly was particularly interested and knowledgeable in anatomy[52] and embryology.[53] This was most likely due to the great influence that Dr. Douglas Stephens had in his career. Dr. Douglas Stephens worked in Melbourne and had a very good reputation because of his studies in anatomy and embryology, chiefly in the urogenital[54] and colorectal areas. Dr. Justin Kelly brought Douglas Stephens' ideas to Boston.

For those readers not familiar with the subject, it is important to note that the main goal in treating an anorectal malformation is not only to create an anus[55] but also to achieve continence. In terms of bowel control, the functional results were very bad in those years. The surgical techniques used were primitive; the surgeons searched for the rectum[56] either through the abdomen (when the rectum

52 The scientific study of the shape and structure of organisms and their parts.

53 Study of the growth and development of organs in animals and human beings.

54 Both the urinary system and the sexual organs, which form together in the developing embryo.

55 Outlet at the terminal end of the anal canal lying in the fold between the buttocks.

56 Terminal portion of the large intestine.

was very high) or through the perineum.[57] This last approach was utilized when the rectum was located near the skin. These were basically blind operations because surgeons did not know the intrinsic anatomy of the malformation. Bowel control was rarely obtained and patients frequently had other complications acquired from the operation, including urinary incontinence and sexual problems.

Dr. Douglas Stephens was the first person to make dissections in cadavers of children born with anorectal malformations. Based on his studies, he wrote a very interesting paper that was published in Australia in 1953. (Ref. 11) He concluded that patients with anorectal malformations have only one important striated sphincter structure[58] (called puborectalis sling), which must be preserved during the repair in order to achieve bowel control. The reason many patients suffered from fecal incontinence after attempted repairs, he asserted, was that the rectum had been pulled down behind the puborectalis sling.

Dr. Stephens described the puborectalis in normal individuals as a muscle that inserted in the pubic bone and surrounded the rectum, inserting in the pubic bone once again. In patients with anorectal malformations, if the rectum was located higher than the puborectalis muscle, then the puborectalis inserted in the pubic

57 Area where the anus normally opens between the anus and the genital organs, including some of the underlying structures.

58 Ridged ring-like muscle which closes a natural orifice or passage

bone, surrounded the posterior urethra[59] (instead of the rectum), reinserting in the pubic bone. With such cases, in order to achieve bowel control, it would be necessary to pass the rectum between the puborectalis and the posterior urethra. (Fig. 1)

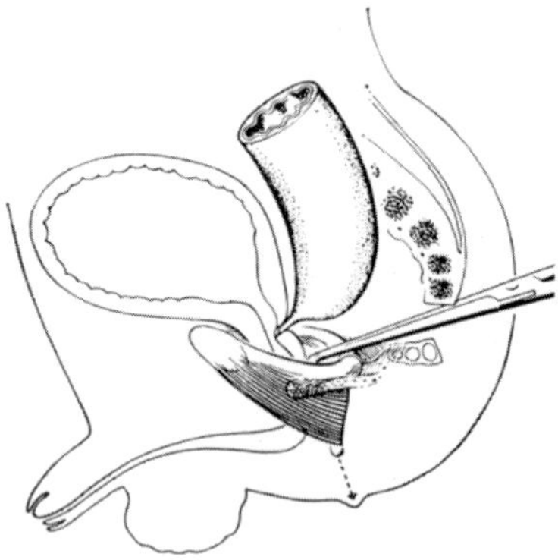

(Fig. 1) Stephen's Repair

To achieve that, Dr. Stephens proposed a special technique in which the patient was situated in prone position[60] while a metallic sound was placed in the urethra to be able to palpate it. A small incision was made in the area of the coccyx[61] granting access to the space above the levator muscle and the puborectalis muscle (which is supposed to be part of the levator mechanism[62]). The rectum should be separated from the urinary tract and, while palpating the metallic sound in the urethra, a tunnel was created between the urethra and the puborectalis muscle. With a right angle clamp, the rectum was then pulled down through the constructed tunnel.

59 The rear of the canal through which urine is discharged from the bladder.

60 Positioned face down.

61 Tailbone.

62 Muscles that elevate an organ or structure.

It was assumed, in the process, that there was no damage done to neighboring structures; yet, the entire procedure was conducted blindly.

In theory, the idea made sense. It was very appealing! Pediatric surgeons all over the world (including me, of course) adopted Dr. Stephens' ideas, operating on these patients while attempting to preserve the puborectalis sling. Some innovators described other techniques but they always attempted to preserve the structure considered key for bowel control. (In fact, even today, many surgeons still try to protect the puborectalis sling.) Dr. Stephens' paper was not well known in the United States (at least not in Boston); therefore, Dr. Justin Kelly shared it with all the surgeons on the staff. Besides those teachings, Dr. Kelly was kind enough to spend extra hours with me, offering me other lessons he had learned from Dr. Stephens.

Now I know that there are many appealing things in life that are not necessarily true. In all of the pediatric surgical meetings discussing anorectal malformations, surgeons would refer to the puborectalis sling but there was only one problem: Only Dr. Stephens alleged to have seen the muscle in post-mortem studies. Nobody else could claim to have done so. We were all "blind believers."

From 1972 until 1980, in Mexico, I worked with anorectal malformations and was able to put together 56 cases (known in those years as high imperforate anus[63]), all of which were approached according to the Douglas Stephens principles. Little by little, throughout those eight years, I introduced minor changes to the Stephens technique. First, I was very uncomfortable working almost blindly through a small incision. Second, I did not feel comfortable passing a right angle clamp behind the urethra, assuming that I was doing it correctly, without really seeing what I was doing.

Gradually, I became more liberal and started extending the midline incision (that was supposed to be extremely small) in the area of the coccyx toward the genitalia.[64] In addition, I decided to use an electrical stimulator because I wanted to see the mysterious puborectalis muscle, once and for all.

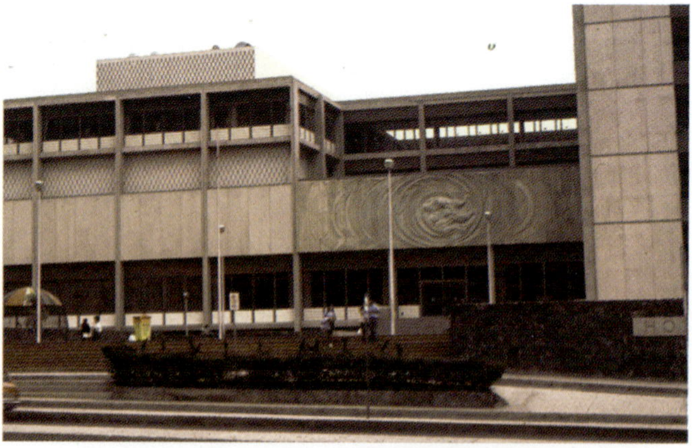

Instituto Nacional de Pediatria (INP), Mexico, DF

SERENDIPITY SMILES

In October of 1971, while making rounds at Children's

63 Congenital absence of the opening of the rectum, having the bowel located high in the pelvis.

64 Reproductive organs, especially the external sex organs.

Hospital Boston, I was paged with a long distance call. It was Dr. Alger Leon-Moreno, the general director of the newest and best-equipped children's hospital in Mexico. "Dr. Alberto Peña? I have an interesting proposition for you. I am pleased to offer you the position of chief of surgery, anesthesia and the intensive care unit at the new hospital here in Mexico City. Are you interested?"

Dr. Alger Leon-Moreno was a military doctor and professor at the Military Medical School yet he could hardly remember me as a student. He heard about me from some friends of mine. I learned another lesson. In those years in Mexico, people complained about the inequality and unfairness of society in general. Many complained that they were unable to achieve academic goals due to unfair politics and/or "lack of contacts." My experience was completely opposite. I was not involved in politics and I had no "contacts" or relatives who helped me.

With this new development, I ended my surgical fellowship (and three year training) at Children's Hospital Boston on December 31st of 1971. In doing so, I immediately became chief of surgery at the Institución Mexicana de Asistencia a la Niñez in Mexico (or INP) *and* professor of pediatric surgery at Universidad Nacional Autonoma de México on January 1st of 1972! Amazingly, and as odd as it may sound, several military pediatric surgeons retired around this same time; therefore, I was also appointed chief of pediatric surgery at the Central Military Hospital!

My day was busy and divided: I worked from 7 a.m. to 11 a.m.

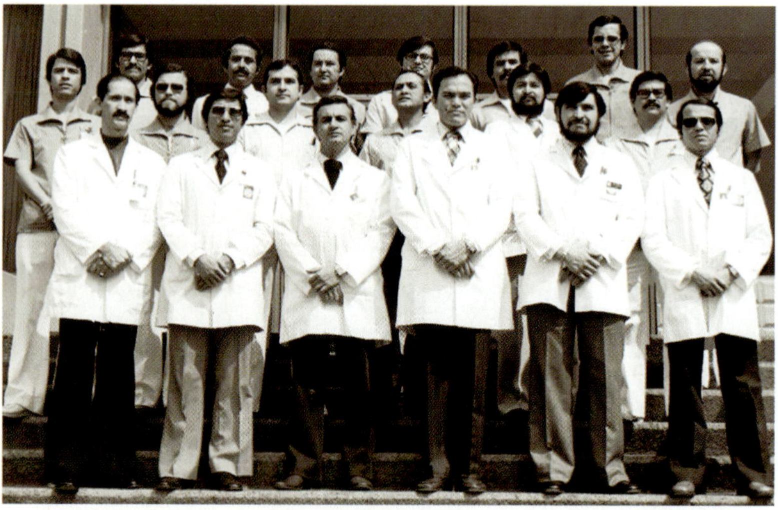

Surgical staff
Front row from left to right: Fernando Villegas, Miguel Vargas, Octavio Ruiz-Speare a virtuoso transplant surgeon and close friend, Alberto Peña, Jaime Olvera and Juan-Manuel Vera; In the back: surgical residents

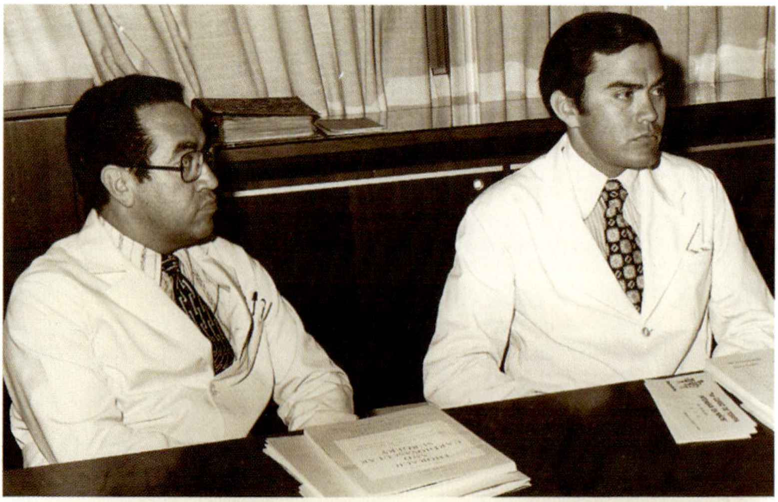

An excellent friend Dr. Eugenio Flammand and Alberto Peña

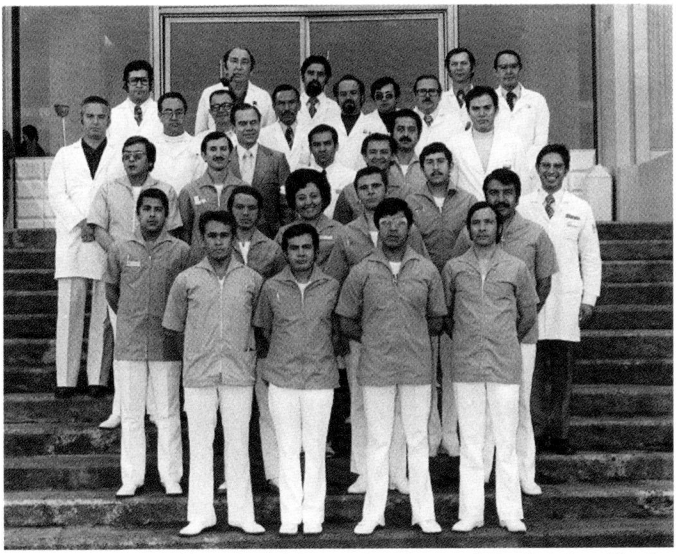

With surgical staff and residents; Institute of Pediatrics Mexico

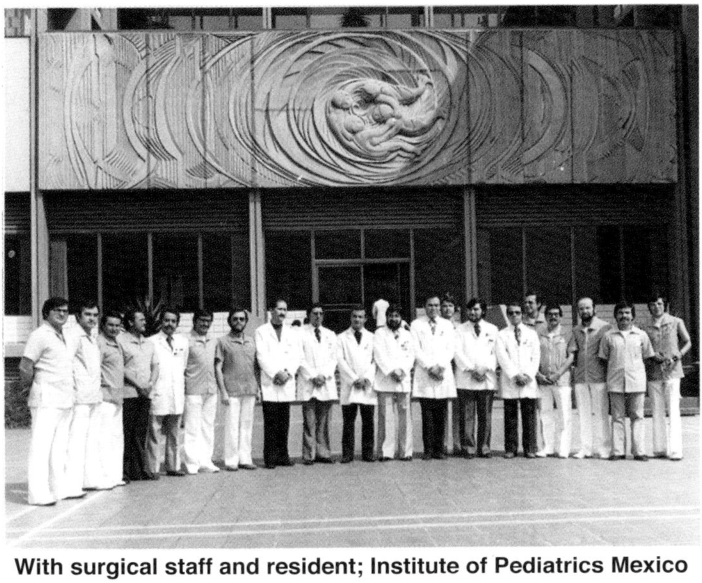

With surgical staff and resident; Institute of Pediatrics Mexico

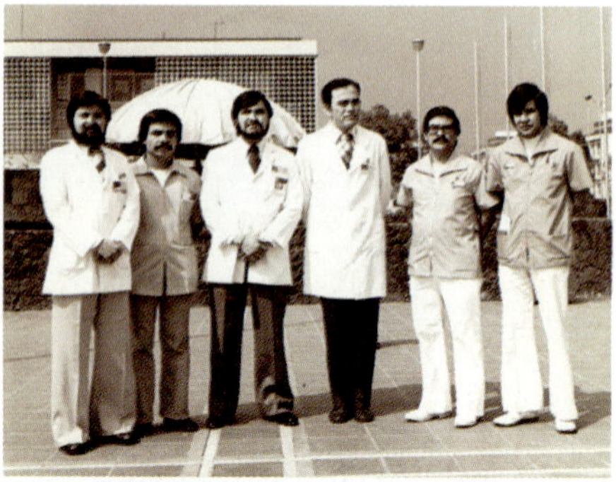

With surgical residents; National Institute of Pediatrics
From left to right: Raul Garnier, Cesar Villatoro, Jamie Olvera, Alberto Peña, Rafael Reyes, Victor Avila

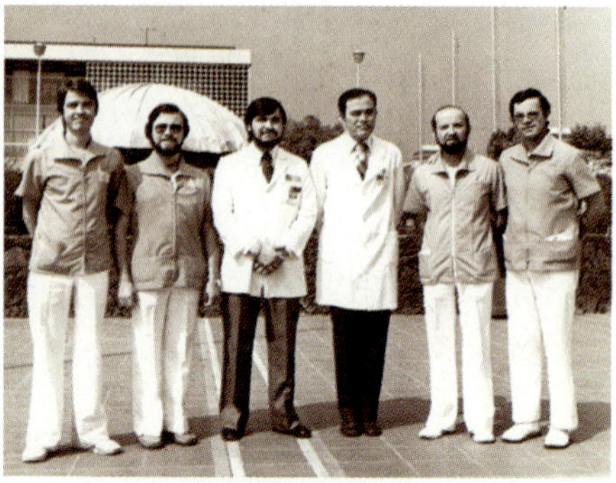

With surgical residents; National Institute of Pediatrics
From left to right: Hugo Staines, Eduardo Teneyuque, Jamie Olvera, Alberto Peña, Camilo Albornoz, Jorge Gonzalez Nava

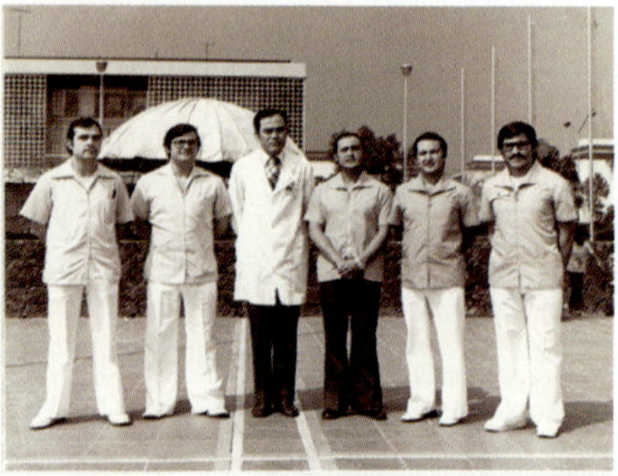

With surgical residents; National Institute of Pediatrics
From left to right: Leopold Torres, Miquel Angel Ojeda, Alberto Peña, Franciso Sosa, Guillermo Gonzalez, Franciso Gonzalez-Prieto

at the Central Military Hospital and the rest of the day at INP. It was indeed overwhelming but fascinating and extremely challenging. At INP, I had four attending pediatric surgeons working for me. I felt an enormous pressure being chief. I was convinced that in order to make a contribution in pediatric surgery, each one of us should focus on studying a specific area. It was impossible to try to be good at everything; so, I invited and encouraged each of the attending surgeons to select one area of interest and work diligently in that subject. They were supposed to read everything they could find, becoming experts on the subject. All of us were to collaborate with the project, referring cases of each specific area to the corresponding surgeon and clinical researcher. This excursion allowed us to operate on a large number of cases and get much more experience in a relatively short period of time—we could gain moral authority and insight while hopefully sparking a creative idea to improve our operations. I told them to feel free to select any subject they wanted and any that they did not, I would accept. Coincidentally, a young surgeon and good friend of mine, Juan Manuel Vera, chose the field of anorectal malformations but then moved to another city. That is why I ended up working in this field. Serendipity at its best!

CONTESTING ANATOMIES

Early on in my operations in patients with high imperforate anus, I used an electrical stimulator and extended the incision distally toward the genitalia, noticing a muscle contraction that I thought was the puborectalis muscle. To make the operation more comfortable and safer, early I decided to make an even longer incision. The retrospective analysis of my 56 cases demonstrated that during the first four years, it was necessary to open the abdomen in 80% of the cases, in order to reach the rectum and pull it down. In the last four years, however, the abdomen was opened in only 20% of the cases. I interpreted these results as evidence that I was becoming more familiar with the anatomy. I was making my incision longer, which made the exposure better; thus, I did not have to open the abdomen so frequently. Furthermore, I discovered that it was possible to divide "the muscle" in the midline to facilitate the separation of the rectum from the urinary tract (in this case, the urethra). I assumed that re-suturing the muscle would not interfere with its function. All of these were modifications to the original Stephens technique.

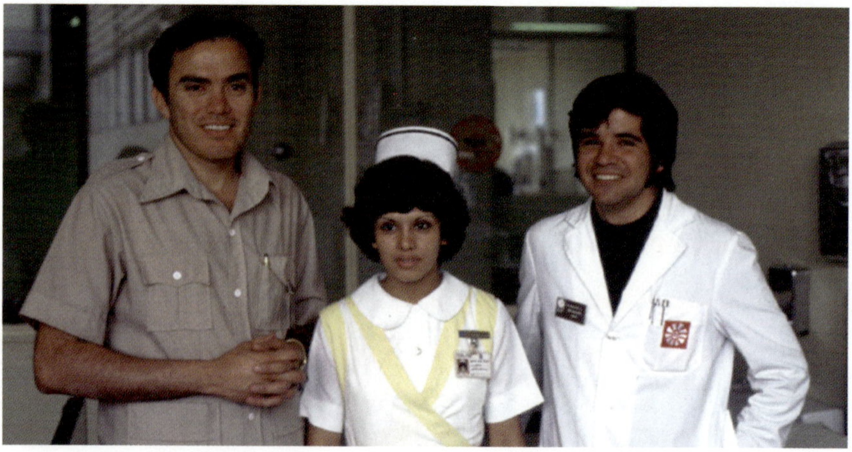

Dr. Alberto Peña, the head nurse, and the Chief Resident Dr. Victor Avila National Institute of Pediatrics, Mexico, 1980

By 1980, I thought it was time to compile a complete analysis and present the findings in an international pediatric surgical meeting. Dr. Victor Avila, chief surgical resident, collaborated with me in the analysis of the series. The paper was accepted for presentation at the annual meeting of the Pacific Association of Pediatric Surgeons in March of 1980 in Colorado Springs. According to the rules, I would only be permitted to present slides and no movies. The contractions of the sphincters were better appreciated when seen in motion during the electrical stimulations. I was not happy.

For that reason, I decided to prepare a three minute long homemade film and smuggle it into the middle of my slide presentation. I carried my projector all the way up to Colorado Springs and my good friend, Dr. Giovanni Porras, was my accomplice in the adventure. When my time came for the presentation, I showed five minutes of slides and, with a high degree of synchronization with Giovanni, three minutes of the movie which dynamically illustrated the contractions of what I presumed was the puborectalis muscle.

In the audience was Dr. Durham Smith, co-author with Douglas Stephens of the foremost book on anorectal malformations. Dr. Durham Smith is a very articulate gentleman and excellent surgeon with a well-deserved international reputation. He commented on my paper, in a very polite way but indicated that what I was showing in the movie was inaccurate. "Dr. Peña, *that* muscle is not the puborectalis muscle. The puborectalis is located much deeper and lower in the pelvis and can only be seen in postmortem studies.

Also, the muscle should be maintained intact, in order to preserve its function."

Exasperated, I could not reply. He was the expert. I was confused, agitated and upset with myself. Now I was much more intrigued to see directly, the anatomic structure that everybody was talking about but nobody had seen during an operation! I was anxious to return to Mexico and explore a patient with an anorectal malformation using a much longer incision, from the middle portion of the sacrum[65] all the way down to the genitalia (in this case, the scrotum[66]). I would use the electrical stimulator and divide every single structure located behind the urethra, in order to describe and document the specific and precise characteristics of that elusive muscle. Dividing everything in the midline, I thought, would not hurt the patient, since I had no knowledge of important nerves or vessels that crossed that area.

The two days that followed my presentation in Colorado Springs I was totally obsessed with the idea of the puborectalis muscle. In conversations with my colleagues, at coffee breaks and cocktails, I was telling everybody what I was planning to do. They patiently and politely listened to me and did not make any comments. Perhaps they felt compassion for me.

On a bus to visit the Air Force Academy, I happened to sit next to Dr. Pieter deVries, a pediatric surgeon from Sacramento,

---

65 Triangular bone at the base of the tailbone.

66 Pouch containing the male reproductive organs (testes).

California. We started talking about my paper and he said that he liked my ideas, which was a great surprise for me. Pieter deVries had a particular interest in the anatomy and embryology of the anorectal malformations. In fact, he conducted experimental studies with chicken embryos. I explained to him what I wanted to do and he seemed enthusiastic, saying that he would like to observe the process. Other surgeons who heard my ideas did not show any interest. But not Pieter. I invited him to Mexico to join me in some of the operations.

THE DIVIDING LINE

On August 10, 1980, Dr. Miguel Vargas and I operated on the first patient using the long incision that eventually was called posterior sagittal approach, looking for the puborectalis muscle. We were extremely meticulous: We made a little cut, stopped and electrically stimulated the area, cut more and continued the

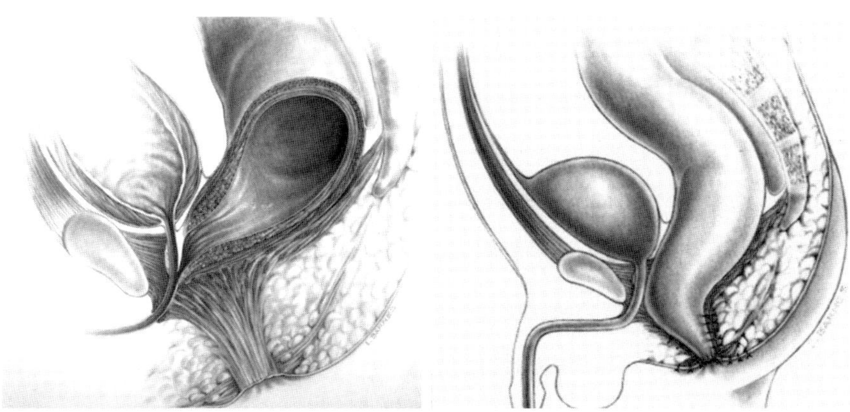

(Fig. 2) Left: The new anatomic concept, 1980; Right: The new repair, 1980

stimulation. We spent several hours searching for a muscle that resembled the structure shown in Dr. Stephens' diagrams. We detected muscle contractions but they did not look at all like the so-called puborectalis muscle. Dr. Vargas and I explored more cases but were unable to detect what we were trying to find.

In the course of those early operations, we identified a specific anatomic pattern of the sphincters. There was no specific structure that resembled the puborectalis; instead, we discerned and documented striated muscle structures that we eventually called parasagittal fibers, muscle complex and levator mechanism. (Fig. 2) Once those structures were identified, the optimal way to reconstruct each malformation became very obvious. (Fig. 2) With the aid of the electrical stimulator, the precise limits of these sphincteral structures were determined. More importantly, though, the rectum could be placed, being sure that it was located within the limits of the sphincters in order for those muscles to play their role in bowel control.

Gradually, I became aware that much more important than the debate about the muscle was that the intrinsic anatomy of the junction of the rectum with the urogenital tract[67] was revealed for the very first time. Due to the wider exposure, Dr. Vargas and I were separating the rectum from the urogenital tract under direct vision. It was now understood just how easy it was to harm the urethra,

67 The urinary system considered together with the organs of reproduction.

the prostate,[68] the seminal vesicles,[69] vas deferens[70] and the nerves that regulate the erection of the penis and bladder function. It was also deduced just how difficult it was to separate these structures blindly, without provoking serious damages. The explanation of so many adolescent patients born and operated with blind or semi-blind procedures suffering from neurogenic bladder,[71] impotence, lack of ejaculation, urethral strictures[72] and retrograde ejaculation[73] was finally uncovered.

We were not conscious of the fact that fully exposing the anatomy of these patients would radically change many concepts. For instance, anorectal malformations were arbitrarily classified in those years, using terms such as "high" and "low," or "high," "intermediate," and "low." Exposing the real anatomy displayed a spectrum of defects. Like in most biological affairs, human beings tend to classify things into groups and categories but I like to think that Mother Nature does not attend these meetings and does not like classifications. She will continue to produce organisms, defects and malformations in spectrums.

The controversy about the anatomy of the sphincters in patients with anorectal malformations prompted me to surgically explore

68 Gland surrounding the bladder neck and urethra in the male, contributing a secretion to the semen.

69 Either of a pair of pouch-like glands situated on each side of the male urinary bladder that secrete seminal fluid and nourish and promote the movement of spermatozoa through the urethra.

70 Main duct of the testicle, through which semen is carried to the urethra, where it ends as the ejaculatory duct.

71 Bladder malfunction secondary to nerve damage.

72 Narrowing of the urethra.

73 Abnormality consisting in ejaculation back into the bladder rather than expelling sperm.

the patients with a much longer incision than was suggested. This not only elucidated the truth about the anatomy but also permitted me to identify many more important anatomic facts crucial to avoid damage during a repair. A good, wide surgical exposure allowed me to create a rational management to correlate the anatomy with the functional prognosis.

*****

In September of 1980, Dr. Jesus Lozoya organized the World Symposium of Pediatric Surgery, in Acapulco, Mexico. Dr. Stephens attended, as well as Dr. Pieter deVries and Dr. Harold Nixon (a prominent pediatric surgeon from London). There was a round table to discuss anorectal malformations and I was asked to present my experience with the Stephens approach. Prior to the meeting in Acapulco, Dr. Pieter deVries visited INP and together, he and I explored more patients with the new, long incision. He even suggested the name "posterior sagittal" for the incision.

At the round table, rather than talk about the Stephens approach, I showed the audience the brand new slides of the intra-operative images from our surgical trials using the posterior sagittal approach. I clearly stated that we divided all the muscle structures located behind the urethra and that we could not see anything that resembled a puborectalis sling. I also showed other structures that were found to be much more interesting—an anatomy that had never been described before. (Fig. 2)

The audience's reaction was mixed. Some doctors, mainly young surgeons, were very enthusiastic. Some of my Mexican colleagues, unfortunately, were upset. Some even went as far as to accuse me of inviting foreign surgeons to do experimental surgery on Mexican children. I shared that with Dr. deVries and he told me that he would invite a certain Mexican surgeon to California to do "experimental surgery" on American children. (Of course, we laughed about that). Eventually, I visited Dr. Pieter deVries in Sacramento and we operated on more cases. Our findings were consistent with those in Mexico. We could not see anything that looked like the puborectalis muscle and again, we defined the limits of the available sphincters in each patient and put the rectum in the right place, giving great hope for better functional results.

Subsequently, Pieter deVries and I went to the next meeting of the Pacific Association of Pediatric Surgeons in Hawaii and presented our results. Our next presentation, with even more experience, was at the American Academy of Pediatrics in New Orleans in 1982. Dr. deVries returned to California and I went back to Mexico to continue our work separately. It seemed that surgeons everywhere were coming around to the idea. Things were looking very promising.

Surprisingly and without any prior discussion about publishing our work, Dr. Pieter deVries took it upon himself to publish the very first paper on the posterior sagittal approach in the *Journal of*

Pediatric Surgery, with his name as the first author and mine as the second! (Ref. 12) Standing up for myself, two months later, I sent another paper to the *Journal of Pediatric Surgery* with my name as the first author and Dr. Pieter deVries as the second author. (Ref. 13) History tells the rest of the story....

SEEING DENIERS

At that point, my professional life became an extraordinary adventure, full of eye-opening episodes, very rewarding events, awards, invitations and accolades—all things I did not plan and actually never struggled to obtain.

INP received a very significant number of cases of anorectal malformations. I wanted to be able to operate on as many patients as possible to learn more about the anatomy of these children, as well as to design the best way to treat them. With that in mind, at the meetings of the Mexican Association of Pediatric Surgeons, I offered to travel to any city within the country and operate on children for free. I offered to pay my traveling expenses and bring all of my surgical instruments and electrical stimulator. Many colleagues were kind enough to invite me to operate on some of their patients, allowing me to collect a significant number of cases in no time at all. I feel a great deal of gratitude toward all of the doctors from Mexico and many other countries for their faith in me.

I was extremely flattered by the request of foreign pediatric surgeons who wanted to witness some of these operations. In order to make those visits more rewarding, I would accumulate several cases to be performed over a period of two or three days. I used to welcome five to ten pediatric surgeons from different countries (mainly the United States). In that short span, we operated on several cases while the surgeons watched directly in the operative field. I called those events "marathons of anorectal malformations."

Since we did not have the extraordinary audiovisual equipment of today, all of the surgeons had to be in the operating room at the same time. Using the new posterior sagittal approach, I showed them the intrinsic anatomy of patients with anorectal malformations. For some time, I was struggling to identify all the anatomic structures

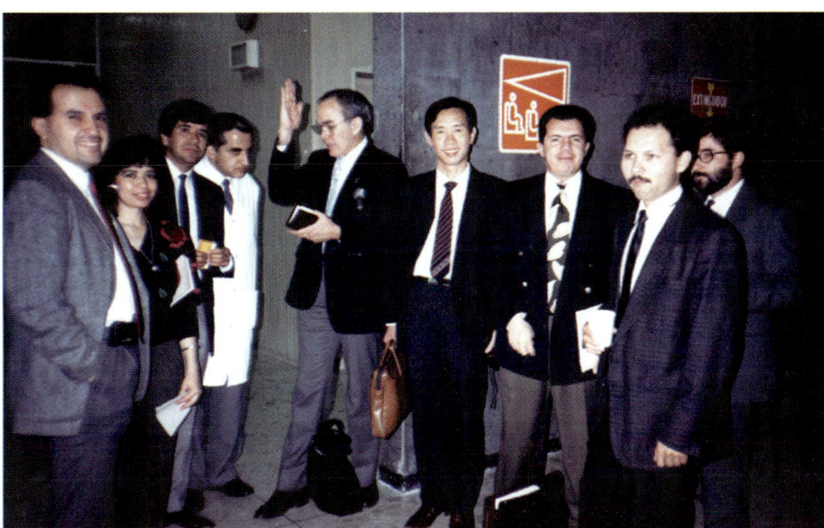

The Preacher
"We must open exactly in the midline, like a book."
From left to right: Dr. Leopoldo Torres, Yolanda Garcia (Dr. Peña's secretary), Dr. Victor Avila, Lazzar Mousali, Alberto Peña, Unidentified, Hector Azuara, Ricardo Sainz, Pastor Fujiyaki

that had been described centuries before in anatomy books. Eventually, I gave up and decided to describe the anatomy in the way it appeared to my assistants and me in reality, not trying to compare it with old textbooks; thus, a new terminology was created. We identified structures such as "parasagittal fibers" and "muscle complex" that were not previously listed in the literature. I stopped using the term puborectalis muscle because I never saw it.

With my multiple trips, I became aware of a certain pattern with the surgeons who invited me. Usually, there was an ambitious young or middle-aged surgeon who promoted the invitation and, frequently, there was a reluctant, skeptical senior surgeon who was not keen about having me. Once acquainted with my young hosts, they shared the troubles they went through to invite me, due to the reluctance and resistance from some of the senior surgeons. That of course is understandable. For a senior surgeon to accept new anatomic concepts, as well as a new way to repair anorectal malformations, implicitly meant that what he had been doing for the previous 30 years was incorrect! There are some extraordinary people, however, for whom seniority does not interfere with their ability to recognize evidence and acknowledge that they were wrong. I had the opportunity to meet senior surgeons who were as enthusiastic and excited about the new developments as if they were very young surgeons (although there were not as many as I would have liked). Disappointingly, there were others who observed the new approach, visualized the real anatomy and continued doing the same old operation for many years, refusing to change their minds. They insisted upon writing articles using the same old terminology and concepts, in spite of their exposure to the real anatomy. These are the "seeing deniers."

AN INVITATION

During the World Symposium of Pediatric Surgery of 1980, Dr. Douglas Stephens was part of the round table in which I presented the long posterior sagittal incision, looking for the puborectalis, showing that the structure was not there (at least not in the way it had been described). I expected Dr. Stephens to comment on my paper but he remained silent.

About two years later I got a phone call from Chicago—it was

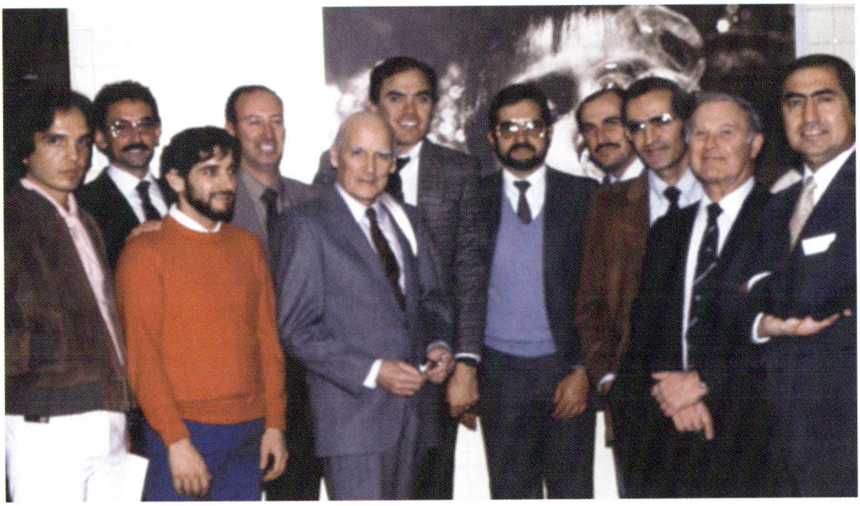

Dr. Stephens' visit to Mexico
From left to right: Jorge Gallego, Unidentified, Froilan Hidalgo, Giovanni Porras, Douglas Stephens, Alberto Peña, Carlos Castro, Pierre Soucy, Unidentified, Stanley Mercer, Unidentified

Dr. Stephens. He told me that he would like to visit my center and see one of those operations. I was very impressed and felt very honored by his request. I put together several cases and welcomed Douglas Stephens to Mexico City.

Dr. Stephens arrived and spent three days with me, having endless conversations and discussions about malformations and embryology. "Alberto, you do not know anything about embryology. You should learn more about it." Pieter deVries was also an embryology-oriented surgeon and he had told me the exact same thing. I felt a bit relieved when Pieter told me that when he discussed embryology with Dr. Stephens, he could not understand him. And when Dr. Stephens was in Mexico, he said the same thing about Pieter. I did not understand either of them so I did not feel too bad.

Even now I recognize that I never excelled in embryology. When I was a medical student I did not like the subject and I still do not like it. I could not see what the professors were describing. I always thought that it was necessary to use a lot of speculation and imagination to understand all the embryology concepts. I still believe that microscopes have reached a limit in what can be seen in the embryologic stages of human life. I confess that I am not an embryology fan and some of my professional experiences reinforce my bias against some embryologic concepts. Whatever the case, I continue to receive many patients who have complex malformations not previously described in the literature. When I describe the grotesque abnormal anatomic findings to surgeons who have been deeply influenced by embryologic concepts, they simply say that it is not embryologically possible; they embraced the embryologic concepts to the point of denying real anatomic facts! My reaction is simple: if an anatomic finding does not match its embryologic explanation, it means that embryologic ideas must be changed.

*****

Prior to his arrival, I read Dr. Stephen's textbook on anorectal malformations, twice. I am used to making notes in the margins of books I read and this time was no exception. With a red pencil and in Spanish, I wrote many rather negative comments about his concepts, even though I knew that his book contained the largest amount of information and best review of anorectal malformations ever written. I admired Dr. Stephens for being the first surgeon who was curious enough to dissect cadavers of children born with these defects. The study of the abnormal anatomy is a mandatory step prior to conceiving the repair of any malformation.

However, I maintain that he came to several erroneous conclusions because he was only able to dissect a few cadavers and, like all humans, he had a preconceived notion about what he was trying to find. The dissection of the cadavers actually did not show anything like the puborectalis depicted in his diagrams. Dr.

Stephens was kind enough to give me a copy of the magnificent photographs of the specimens that he studied in cadavers. The anatomy shown in these pictures resembles more of what I saw in my operations; yet, Dr. Stephens persisted in depicting the puborectalis muscle. Like many others, I believe:

Our eyes may see only what we want to see.

In addition, anorectal malformations are represented by a wide spectrum of defects. Patients with anorectal malformations usually do not die. Only those with severe associated defects die. By definition, I believe these patients are not typical of the spectrum of anorectal malformations and perhaps that is another reason why Dr. Stephens was wrong about the anatomy and surgical treatment of these malformations. I had the opportunity to discuss many of my ideas with him and consider myself his friend. He is an admirable individual. We still disagree.

One afternoon during Dr. Stephens' visit, I had some bureaucratic work to do in the administrative offices and I asked him to wait for me in my office. So, Dr. Stephens sat at my desk. He looked at my bookshelf, found his book and found all my comments written in Spanish with a red pencil. Dr. Stephens could not understand any of them. He opened my office door and patiently waited until one of my surgical residents passed. "Excuse me. Can I ask you a favor?"

"Of course, Sir," the resident said courteously.

"Please, I'm having trouble with this. Can you translate this for me?"

The intimidated resident read my aggressive comments, his

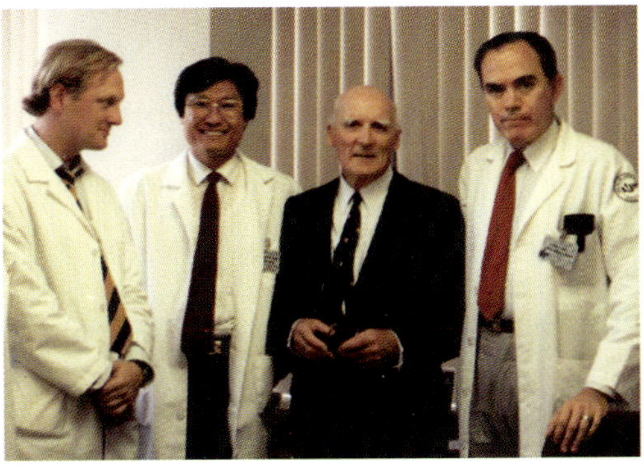

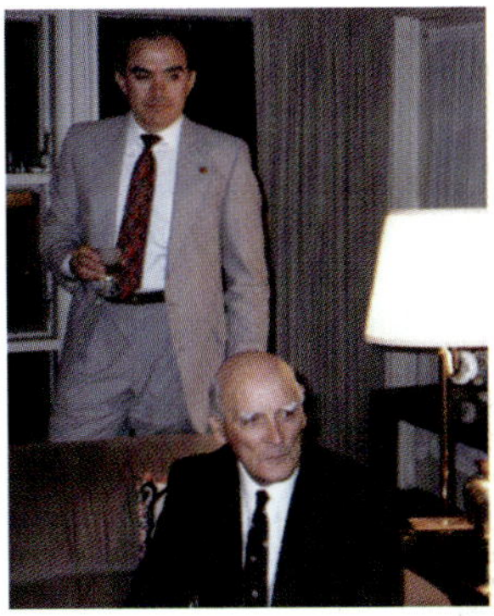

On the left, Schneider Children's Hospital, Long Island N.Y.
From left to right: Henrik Hedlund, Dr. Wang, Douglas Stephens, Alberto Peña
On the right, Alberto Peña, and Douglas Stephens in Long Island N.Y.

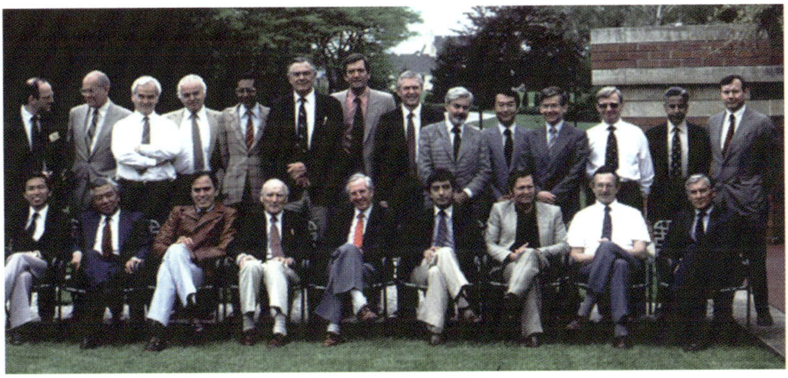

Wingspread Meeting
Seated from left to right: Dr. Ikeda, Dr. Yokohama, Alberto Peña, Douglas Stephens, Durham Smith, Nicolas Martin-del-Campo, Alex Holschneider, Sydney Cywes, John Raffensperger; Standing up: Stephen Dolgin, Dr. Donellan, Freeman, Peter Kottmeier, Subir Chaterjee, Pieter de Vries, David Gough, Dale Johnson, Barry Shandling, Unidentified, Lois Scharli, Harold Nixon, Unidentified, Jack Templeton

face turned pale and he very politely replied, "Dr. Peña wrote that he agrees with everything in your book."

Later, Dr. Stephens scrubbed in with me and I showed him directly the anatomic findings of our patients. He made no comments.

Dr. Stephens returned to Chicago and soon after, together with Dr. Durham Smith, organized a special meeting in Wisconsin at a residence known as Wingspread (designed by Frank Lloyd Wright). He invited about 20 doctors from all over the world who demonstrated particular interests in anorectal malformations. We spent three days there discussing classification and management of these malformations. I felt like Dr. Stephens and Dr. Smith were looking for a consensus, a kind of compromise between old concepts and new ones. As a consequence, the old classification of anorectal malformation (elaborated by Doctors Stephens and Smith in Melbourne, Australia) was changed to the Wingspread Classification. During that meeting, I was the eternal opponent to most of the present pediatric surgeons. Even though there was significant progress compared to the old one, I did not agree with the final classification.

In May 2005, Dr. Stephens again, with Dr. Durham Smith and Dr. Alexander Holschneider from Cologne, Germany, organized another meeting. At long last, the classification, known as the Krickenbeck Classification or International Classification, looked much more like the one that I always proposed.

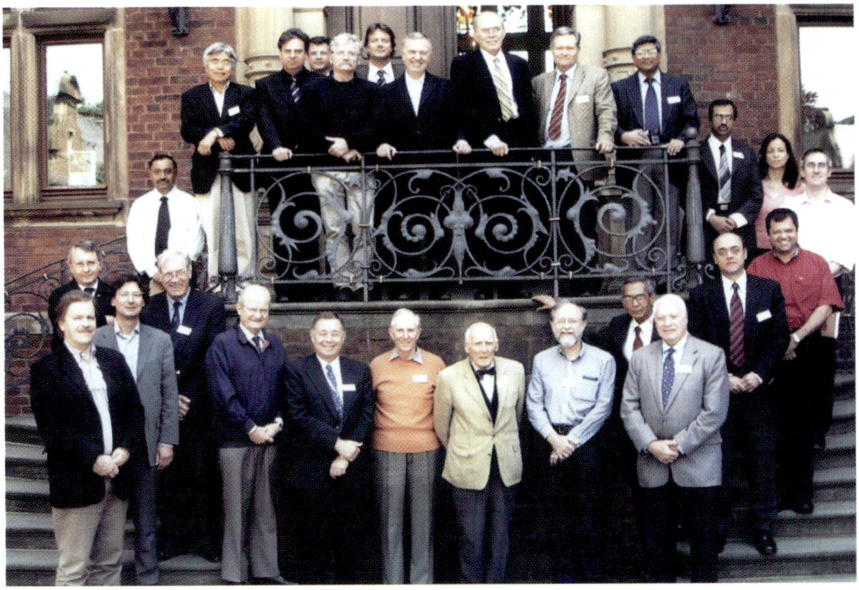

Krickenbeck Meeting
Top row from left to right: Naomi Iwai, Giuseppe Martucello, Unidentified, Dieter Kluth, Thomas Boemers, Keith Georgeson, Alberto Peña, Alex Holschneider, Devendra Gupta; Front row left to right: Risto Rintala, Reinhold Engelskirchen, Benno Ure, Samuel Moore, Michael Davies, Arnold Coran, Durham Smith, Douglas Stephens, John Hutson, Subir Chaterjee, Jay Grosfeld; On the stairs left side: Sudipta Sen; On the stairs right side: Sabine Grashoff, V. Sripathi, and Feilin Murphy

ANOTHER RATIONAL APPROACH

Cloacae are malformations occurring in females. Rather than having a urethra, vagina and rectum, these girls are born with a single orifice that communicates through a single channel that trifurcates into a rectum, vagina and urethra. Prior to 1982, there was not an established approach to repair cloacae. Many of these patients died or grew up with very serious problems, including fecal and urinary incontinence, as well as a very poor sexual life. Dr. Hardy Hendren had the largest experience on the subject. (Ref. 14-16) I

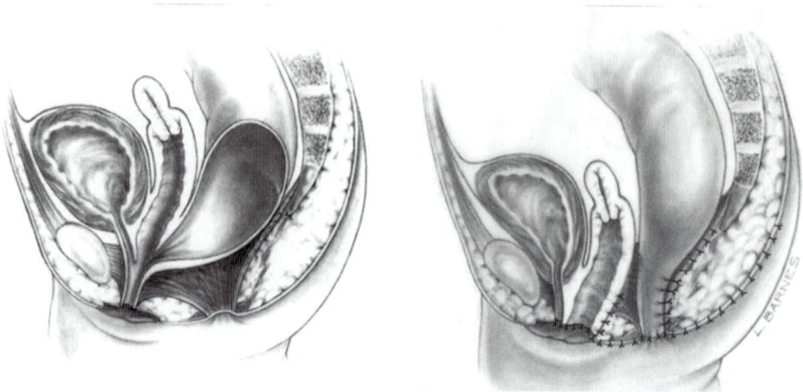

(Fig. 3) Left: Diagram of a cloaca; Right: Diagram of a repaired cloaca

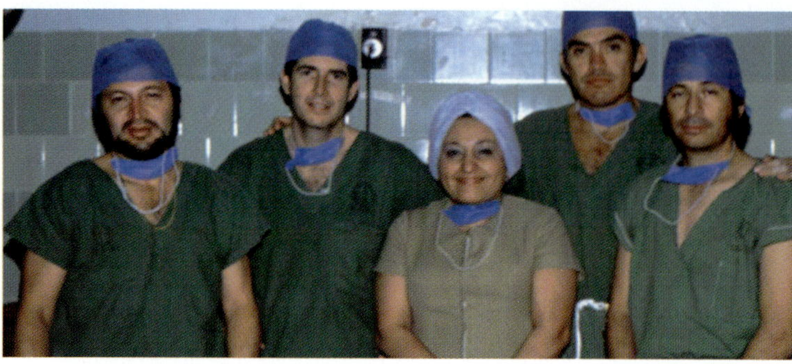

The first cloaca repair done using the "new" approach
From left to right: Raul Garnier, Marshall Schwartz, Maricela Zarate, Alberto Peña, Ulises Garza, University Hospital, Monterrey, Mexico

could not have predicted that the posterior sagittal approach would represent the ideal way to reconstruct this complex abnormality. (Fig. 3)

I was invited to operate on one of these cases for the first time in Monterrey, in the north of Mexico, by one of my ex-surgical residents, Dr. Maricela Zarate. Coincidentally, Dr. Marshall Schwartz (a renowned pediatric surgeon from Galveston, Texas) was visiting me in Mexico and I invited him to join us for the first cloaca repair using the new approach. Fortunately, that patient happened to belong to what is now known as the "benign" side of the spectrum of cloacae. I was lucky—it was a cloaca that now I consider relatively easy to repair. I like to say:

God protects innocence.

That little girl is now a young lady with urinary control, bowel control and is sexually active. The fact that I was confronted with a cloaca with benign anatomy encouraged me to continue. If I had been exposed to a complex cloaca (that are today referred to me) perhaps I would have stopped operating on such cases. The repair of cloacae has always been very interesting; every time I operate on one of these patients, I learn a new lesson. I am up to almost 500 cloaca cases operated—still counting and still learning.

History shows that the field of anorectal malformations was rather abandoned through many years. The explanation may reside in the fact that it is not an elegant subspecialty because it deals with stool, urine and sex—all relatively awkward concepts to talk about socially. Modern science and technology were almost never applied to this particular field. This is sad but at the time it represented a great prospect to be able make a contribution with a relatively minor effort. What began as a burning curiosity for me to observe anatomic structures that were subjects of controversy had unexpectedly wonderful, rewarding implications, benefiting many children. In any human activity, while looking for the truth, people know where they started but cannot predict where they will end.

A SEARCH FOR SUCCESS

Most of the techniques used to correct congenital malformations of the gastrointestinal tract[74] were conceived, described and performed by bold, brave, ambitious surgeons mostly during the second half of the nineteenth century and the first half of the twentieth century. To do that, these pioneers had to go through three main steps: 1) to know and understand the normal anatomy 2) to learn about the anatomic abnormality (typically in the autopsy room) and 3) to conceive a feasible repair. Suddenly, patients originally condemned to die, survived and the surgeon, brave enough to try and succeed first, became a kind of celebrity. Interestingly, in the field of anorectal malformations, until 1980 step number two was missing.

The techniques originally described to correct malformations are not much unlike those used now. Extraordinarily different, though, are the great technologic advances that allow more accurate diagnosis, safer anesthesia techniques, pulmonary support, metabolic support, antibiotic therapy, intensive care, and perioperative technology. The same type of operations that were done by the pioneers are now performed under better circumstances, in a quiet environment, with excellent visualization of the operative field, meticulous hemostasis, delicate instruments

74 Part of the digestive system consisting of the stomach, small intestine and large intestine.

and sutures and lately, with minimally invasive procedures. In terms of survival and recuperation, the results of these operations, of course, are much better.

RECORDING THE RESULTS

With the first patient to receive the posterior sagittal approach in August of 1980, we identified the limits of the sphincter and located the rectum within the limits of the sphincter, expecting that all the patients would be completely fecally continent. To that, I can say that we were partially right. Very soon, I was faced with the most significant lesson: this is a spectrum of defects.

On the good side of the spectrum, are patients with favorable anatomies. If repaired correctly, they behave like normal or almost normal children. On the bad side of the spectrum, there are patients born with serious anatomic deficiencies that make it impossible to develop bowel and urinary control. Fortunately, the majority of patients (about 75%) belong to the good side of the spectrum. It is important to note that the operations required to repair these malformations are technically demanding and require sensitivity plus a delicate technique. When patients born with good functional prognoses type of defects receive a technically deficient repair, they will endure permanent sequelae (mainly fecal incontinence). This is very awful and unfortunately happens very often.

I have been confronted with patients who underwent operations performed with blind and semi-blind techniques, suffering from serious sequelae. I re-explored as many of those patients as possible and surveyed how many mistakes and complications happened when these operations were performed blindly. I repaired these problems and many of the patients had very rewarding results. Others did not. I found that many patients with previous operations were left with the rectum completely mislocated. I replaced the rectum and by doing so I expected all of them to regain bowel continence but found that only about half of them did so. There were many other factors that had to be analyzed. Through all these years, I learned that human beings tend to be extremely simplistic in their way of reasoning. Doctors frequently try to cheat Mother Nature only to learn that they have to work much harder and think much deeper about the complexity of the biological phenomenon.

Through the years, I learned to suspect and identify most of the associated defects[75] that these patients have: 30% of them have an orthopaedic defect,[76] 25% have a neurosurgical condition,[77] 10% of them a cardiovascular malformation[78] and 50% have urologic problems. Doctors cannot ignore these problems; rather, they must suspect them in order to diagnose for early treatment to avoid future sequelae. It is extremely important to suspect something in order to make a correct diagnosis. From August of 1980, until the moment of writing this, I have operated on over 2000 patients with anorectal

75 Congenital malformations usually occurring and related to other defects.

76 Problems that develop in the bones, joints and ligaments of the human body. Mainly spinal problems in these cases.

77 Problems with any part of the nervous system.

78 Defects of the heart and blood vessels.

malformations. The information obtained has been documented in over 150 publications and numerous book chapters...I am still learning.

I was fortunate enough to make notes and records of the anatomic details as well as the associated defects and numerous events that occurred during the operations performed since 1980. Eventually, those records became a larger document and now are included in a valuable database that I treasure. In addition, I attempted to follow each one of my patients, which proved to be an extremely complicated, time consuming but invaluable task. Pediatric surgeons operate on children and it is extremely important to understand the long-term benefits and negative consequences of operations. I strongly recommend to all pediatric surgeons to stay in contact with their patients for as long as possible, particularly those ailing from serious congenital malformations. This is the best way to learn and contribute to pediatric surgery.

I am convinced that in order to make a contribution in medicine or surgery, it is necessary to work hard and focus on a specific problem. In turn, this strategy raises more and more fascinating questions. It is like pulling an endless string. Very soon in the process, it is determined that it is very complicated to progress without collaborating with other specialized clinicians and basic scientists. This explains why, while working in New York, I conceived the idea of creating a multidisciplinary center dedicated to the study, treatment, and advancement in the management of

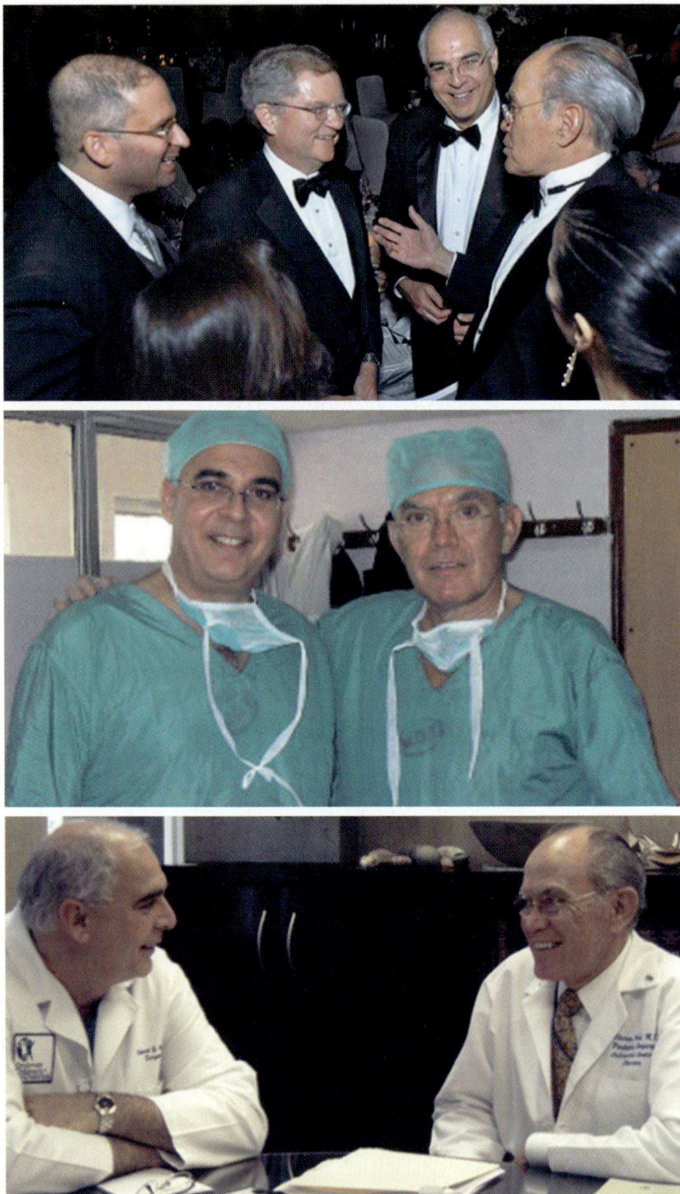

Top: Dr. Levitt, Mr. Anderson, Richard Azizkhan, Dr. Peña; Middle and Bottom: Dr. Peña with Dr. Azizkhan, Surgeon-in-Chief with vision, Cincinnati Children's Hospital

colorectal problems and the associated conditions in children. For this, it is necessary to have visionary leaders, working in prominent institutions with a strong infrastructure, to guarantee a secure and solid future. Dr. Marc Levitt, my partner of 19 years, played a key role to achieve this. He and I presented the idea to several institutions within the US, obtaining varied responses. Dr. Richard Azizkahn and Mr. James Anderson, surgeon-in-chief and CEO of Cincinnati Children's Hospital (respectively) accepted and fully supported our idea. And, in July of 2005, we created the Colorectal Center for Children at Cincinnati Children's Hospital Medical Center. So far, the achievements of the Center are much better than we expected.

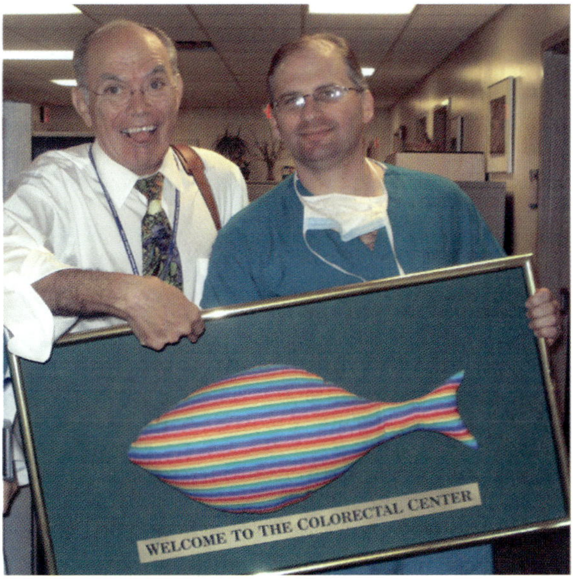

With a loyal collaborator and friend Dr. Marc Levitt

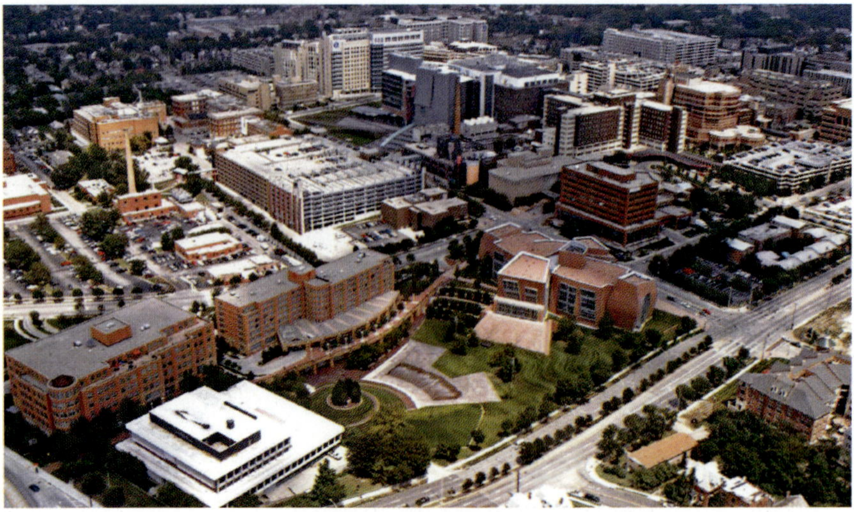

Cincinnati Children's Hospital Medical Center

A GREAT CHALLENGE

It is extremely important to emphasize that the biggest challenge accompanying the repair of congenital malformations remains: functional sequelae. To conceive and apply a surgical technique to repair a malformation for the first time, no doubt, requires imagination, boldness, ambition and skills. Compared with the enormous challenge of dealing with functional sequelae, this seems an easy task. A surgeon can now repair an esophageal atresia[79] safely but does not know what to do about the dysmotility[80] of the esophagus[81] that will trouble the patient. A surgeon can safely repair a diaphragmatic hernia[82] but is still challenged and puzzled

79 Birth defect in which the tube connecting the mouth to the stomach (esophagus) is segmented and closed.

80 Ability to move spontaneously and independently.

81 Tube that connects the mouth with the stomach.

82 Hernia through the diaphragm.

by the persistent problem of pulmonary hypertension[83] that the patient must endure.

In the field of anorectal malformations, patients born with "benign" defects can have almost normal lives as a result of a good surgical technique. On the other hand, surgeons can repair the anatomy of patients born with very serious anatomic deficiencies but cannot completely reestablish their function. At least 25% of all children born with an anorectal malformation will suffer from a lack of bowel control. This is a great challenge.

After almost 30 years of working in this field, the fight continues on several fronts:

Trying to improve surgical techniques, mainly in cases of complex malformations, attempting to achieve better functional results.

Training as many pediatric surgeons as possible throughout the world to avoid preventable catastrophic complications and surgical misadventures that departs serious functional sequelae in children born with malformations with potential for bowel and urinary control.

Implementing medical rehabilitation programs aimed to keep the patients artificially clean of stool and dry of urine, in order to avoid discrimination and distress. To that end, a special program called Bowel Management Program has been created. This program produces a dramatic improvement in the lives of children with fecal

83 Abnormally high blood pressure in the arteries of the lungs, making the right side of the heart work harder than normal.

incontinence.

Aside from legal and ethical concerns, it is foreseeable that prenatal[84] diagnoses will progress enough to make early accurate diagnoses of these defects, giving parents alternatives including the possibility of interrupting the pregnancy.

Much later in the future, geneticists will probably be able to manipulate genetic material to avoid hereditary or predisposed defects altogether.

*****

I feel extremely honored to be part of this extraordinary experience. I successfully operated on many children who now enjoy normal or almost normal life. I have had the opportunity to learn about their happy lives as adults and I have lived long enough to be able to operate on the children of my patients. I have also suffered with all of those patients who I operated on and was unable to give a good quality of life due to the severity of their functional sequelae.

HIDDEN MERIT

Throughout my life I was offered many flattering remarks and received demonstrations of admiration related with my contribution to the field. Mostly, it came from very good loyal friends and relatives; some came from doctors or persons I never

84 Existing or occurring before birth.

met. Although extremely rare, I also heard some rather negative comments.

A group of friends and relatives invited me to express my personal opinion about the merit of my contributions. (An awkward task, to say the least.) I thought about it and came to a conclusion. I considerably enjoyed every minute of my career but the discovery and description of the intrinsic anatomy of the spectrum of anorectal malformations, conceptually and intellectually, is extremely simplistic. It did not require any effort on my part; therefore, I do not see any merit in it. On the other hand, I consider the therapeutic implications and benefits received by many children to be very significant. But again, it did not require any effort on my behalf.

There is merit, however, in an area that is rarely recognized. This is a valuable message for young doctors, particularly those who were born and work in developing countries. To have an original idea has no merit because it does not require any effort. The merit resides in believing in your own observation and having the tenacity to defend your concept, the intellectual honesty to identify your limitations and to present and defend your concepts in front of a forum of experts and pundits with differing ideas on the subject.

To be an academic surgeon in an institution or a country that does not reward academicism is not easy. The great majority of children's hospitals in developing countries are public institutions and doctors' salaries are very low. In order for the doctors to earn enough money to provide for the family's basic needs, it is necessary for them to work extra hours in private institutions. Books, slides, videos, movies, meetings, reprints and journals must be paid for out of the doctors' pockets. Moreover, corruption, politicking, environmental deterioration and unfavorable living conditions all conspire against an academic career. My recognition goes to all those professionals who live under trying, complex circumstances and manage to devote part of their mental energy and meager resources to conceive better ways to operate on children. Being able to concentrate on ideas and projects without immediate gratification, while overcoming all these obstacles in the process, is meritorious.

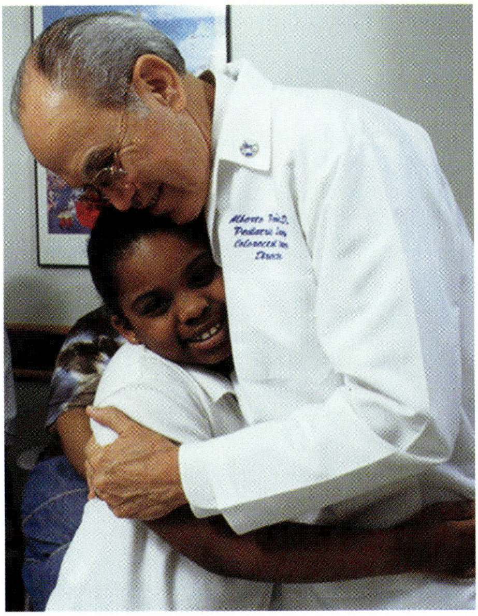

THE RELATIONSHIP WITH PATIENTS AND PARENTS

The practice of medicine is becoming more and more bureaucratically controlled. Doctors are told that patients do not belong to them but to the hospital. In fact, there are rules related with the ownership of the medical records and personal information. Years ago, the doctor maintained *his* patients as well as their medical records. The doctor would analyze the results of his treatments, communicate with the patients directly and he would consider them *his* patients. Reciprocally, patients used to talk about *their* doctor. That feeling is dangerously disappearing. It is becoming more complicated for patients to select their doctors.

As medicine and surgery continue to "progress" and the litigations and administrative pressures increase, hopefully, the essence of the relationship between doctor and patient will remain a human, emotional one, full of faith, confidence and friendship. Without these ingredients, perhaps it is not worth practicing medicine. Unfortunately, some physicians, perhaps unintentionally, promote the rather cold, impersonal, antagonistic, contractual relationship with their patients.

I have observed events that can be considered "bad symptoms" in terms of the doctor-patient relationship. During a pediatric surgical meeting, I watched a presentation on "the financial benefits of post-operative phone follow-up in pediatric surgery" and was alarmed by the complacency of the audience. I cannot stop wondering if the paradigm is changing.

Pediatric surgeons have a very powerful influence on an individual's quality of life that could reach into the next 75 years. It is fascinating to follow-up with patients over this time. This long-term analysis reveals the benefits and complications of operations. It is imperative for surgeons to follow patients for as long as possible and to the best of their abilities. Some surgeons consider a job completed when the patient recovers from the operation. They refer the patient back to the pediatrician and the pediatrician conducts the follow-up. What the long-term analysis provides is invaluable information that could be applied in practice and preserved for others to learn.

Nothing is more rewarding than becoming emotionally involved with patients. The desire to do better work derives from positive feedback. There is great satisfaction in reading a letter from a patient who was operated on as a newborn, wanting to share her happiness because she graduated from the university, got married and had a child! Equally important is the feedback of witnessing the pain and anguish of a patient and his family as a result of a poor operation. Though heartbreaking, this represents a major motivation to search for better ways to treat patients.

It takes a long time to learn what to do, but it takes much longer to learn what not to do.

*****

The surgeon's dialogue is established with the patient, with the parents and frequently involves the grandparents. The terms used, as well as the content of the conversation, change completely depending on the patient's age. Doctors should be aware of the mentality of each age group in order to establish a real communication and dialogue with them. Conversations must also differ depending on the cultural background of the family. This means that the doctor must be trained to deal with each of these specific circumstances on an individual basis.

A four-year-old child needing an appendectomy[85] does not

85 Surgical removal of the appendix.

want to know the meaning of the word. He just wants to know if the procedure is going to hurt and if Mommy is going to be next to him. A school age child may understand that her abdomen will be opened but it must be explained that she is not going to feel a thing because she will be sleeping. A teenager may understand that it is better to do the operation now, before the appendix[86] ruptures and the problem gets worse. It is unnecessary to provide gratuitous and confusing information.

A pediatric surgeon must try to identify the mentality, worries, concerns and fears of his little patients. A common fear in school age children is the idea that they will wake up in the middle of an operation. The conversation with a 14-year-old female patient with lower abdominal pain may be complicated because of the potential gynecologic[87] implications involving the possibilities of cysts torsions, or sexually related conditions, such as pregnancy or venereal diseases. All of these are complicated topics to discuss at such a sensitive transitional age, in an ever-changing, multicultural and multi-religious society. Dialogues with the parents and grandparents, on the other hand, must be more informative since they will give permission to operate on the child. A great deal of sensitivity is expected from the doctor confronted with such scenarios.

*****

86 The worm-shaped pouch attached to the junction of the small and large intestines.

87 Pertaining to the study of diseases of the female reproductive organs and the breasts (gynecology).

A recurring question is how much information should be provided to the patient and the family. Current literature is talking more in favor of giving as much information as possible although, unfortunately, the main motivation seems to be legalistic. Information originally geared to help patients and families understand a treatment to be provided, now seems to be aimed to protect the doctor and the institution in the event of a medico-legal problem. Although I agree with the idea of giving the patients and families as much information as they require, I do not agree with the trend of making such information a legally oriented process. I also do not believe in the idea that the information should be equal for everybody.

I remember an uneducated, poor mother listening to my explanation of a complex operation that I was going to perform on her son. This operation was going to improve his life but certainly was not going to avoid significant sequela—it was a lengthy and potentially risky procedure. I was young and I was explaining everything in great detail. The mother was holding my hands tightly and right after I finished my extensive explanation, she looked at me, "But my son is going to be alright, right?" I realized that she actually did not listen to what I said. All she wanted to hear from me is that her son was going to be all right. And that is what I told her.

Of course, parents have common sense and intuition and they

understand the most important aspects of what will be done to their children. Some parents are extremely educated and intellectual, some of them are even doctors and, according to their background, they demand and expect certain consistent, comprehensive information about what is happening. Others require and expect a more simplified explanation. And, as odd as it may sound, another group actually does not want to hear an explanation at all. They would rather have support, trusting the doctor's proficiency.

I am basically against the formulaic cliche-type of explanation given in an indiscriminate manner to *all* parents of *all* children, despite of their background, level of education, sensitivity and curiosity. I have seen many young surgeons upsetting parents by giving them "technically correct information" about an operation. The first problem is that the surgeons adopt a technical jargon that they think is cool, professional and appropriate. They speak in a fast, technically oriented, sophisticated, intellectually elegant way, regardless of the family. The parents may or may not understand what is said; they may feel intimidated and afraid to ask questions. This same speech is repeated to all kinds of parents. Even when the surgeon complies with the correct protocol, the parents actually do not comprehend one word; instead, they perceive the doctor as a distant figure, performing his duty, displaying no authentic interest in their child. They feel that the doctor is, in some way, trying to protect himself.

*****

Besides security, there are many reasons why passengers of a commercial airliner are not allowed to enter the cockpit. The passengers are unable to hear what the pilots are discussing—allowing the passengers to participate in the conversation would be chaotic. For instance, passengers might panic without a real concern when they hear the captain say, "I think we made a mistake." Without the technical knowledge, the passengers cannot put that statement into proper context. What would happen if the captain came out every hour and provided information about navigational concerns, asking for opinions about what to do?

Something similar happens when surgeons offer excessive amounts of unsolicited, indigestible information to a patient or their parents, expecting them to decide the best course of action. Parents understand that there are no guarantees; so, it is not adequate to share *all* of the hesitations and concerns that pass through a doctor's mind.

Desperate and totally confused, many times the parents reach out, "If he was your son what would you do?" Doctors must remember that the parents of a child with a malformation are looking for help and help can only come from someone perceived as being knowledgeable, mature, compassionate and skilled. Someone with moral authority. Someone with professionalism and the knowledge of the surgical techniques capable of solving their

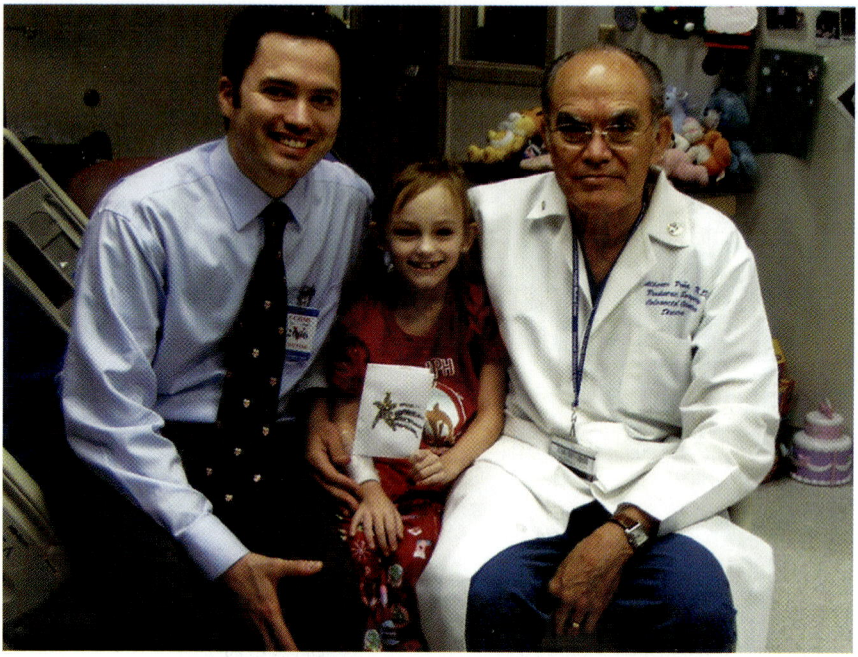

Above: Dr. Victor Peña, Molly, and Alberto Peña

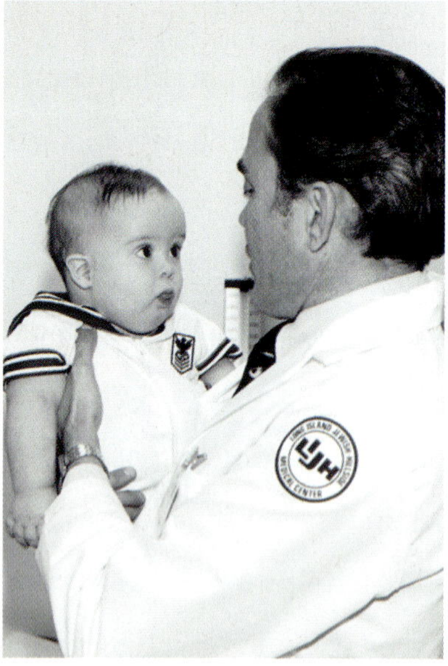

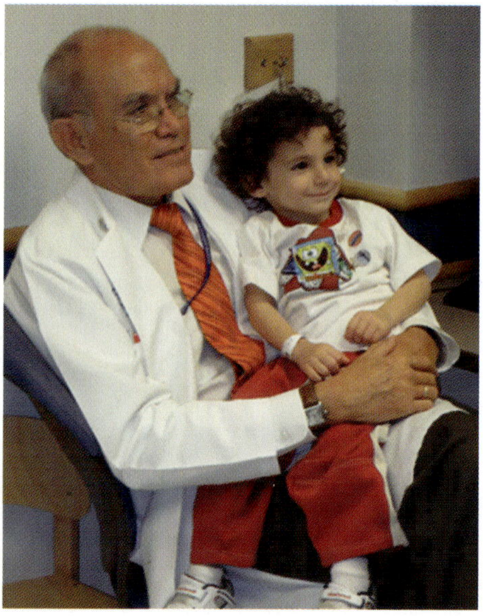

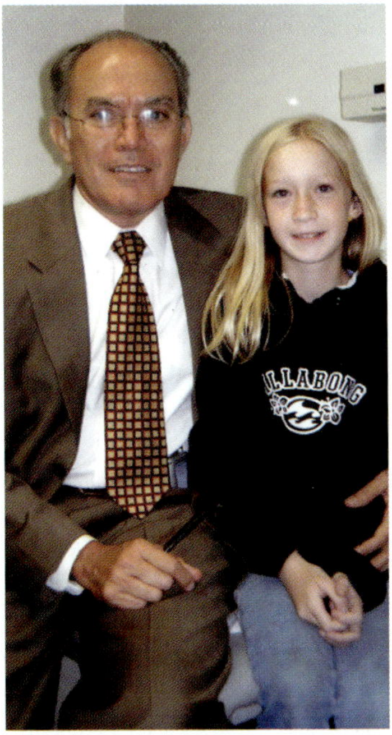

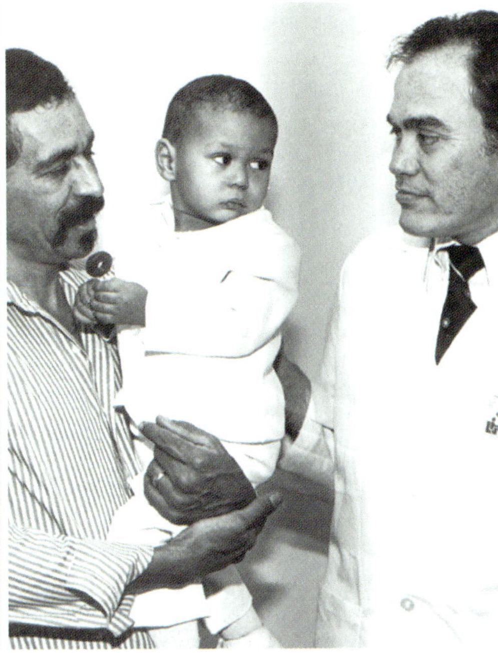

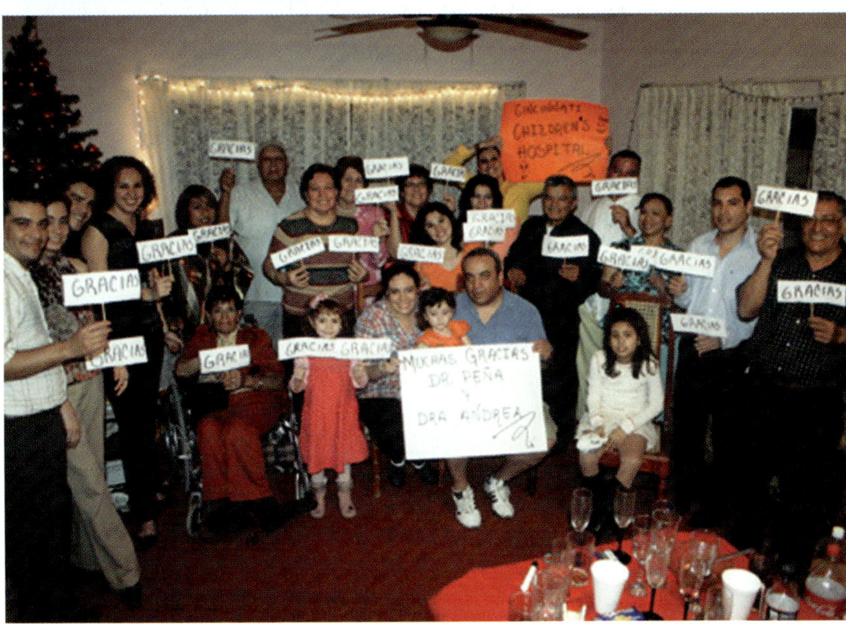
GRACIAS
MUCHAS GRACIAS
DR. PEÑA
Y
DRA ANDREA

child's problem. When parents come for help, it is because they think that they have found that kind of person. This must be taken as a serious responsibility.

*****

Some parents arrive for the first consultation and they already appear angry. They are angry with life, with the world and they are angry with society. They are upset because they were sent a child with a congenital defect and they think they do not deserve that. Sometimes this is a very successful couple that has always planned everything in a rational way and they expect a successful outcome in everything they do, including having children. Furthermore, they are accustomed to finding an answer and a solution for every crisis they encounter.

When there is a problem in a large company, a specific expert or consultant is called to solve the problem, whatever the cost. They bring in the right expert from wherever he is and they expect guaranteed solutions. In medicine things are slightly different. Surgeons sometimes perform operations that restore the patient to a basically normal life but many other times, they repair a malformation that leaves the patient with serious sequela, preventing a reintegration into a completely normal life. Surgeons are obligated to tell the parents, possibly making them angrier.

*****

Parents sometimes go "shopping" from clinic to clinic, from surgeon to surgeon, comparing notes and intentionally not disclosing that they already heard several previous opinions. They are looking for inconsistencies. In fact, when they find those inconsistencies, they do not trust the surgeons. When confronted with these situations, the first principle is not to respond to the parents' aggressive attitudes. Keep in mind, regardless of their hostile disposition, they are suffering human beings passing through one of the most harrowing times of their lives. Very few things in life are as distressing as having a child with a very serious ailment. Even when they look powerful, knowledgeable and aggressive, actually, hidden inside are two agonizing souls requiring support. They check statistics and notes and they ask sophisticated questions. Rather than responding to their attitude and harsh language, it is integral to try to aid them, not only professionally but also emotionally. Doctors are not there to quarrel with parents. They are there to help.

A doctor could volunteer to the parents, "I am going to give you some advice as a father, not as a doctor. Look for two or three of what you think are the best trained and experienced surgeons to care for your child. Have a few words with them and determine with whom you feel more empathy and whom you trust. Try to relax. Let the surgeon take care of your child. Do not interfere. After all, you are dealing with the top doctors in the country. If you do not think that the surgeon is your best option, go to another place but once you have reached that place put your confidence and trust with that person and let them work." Eventually, they will appreciate the advice. After all, that is what surgeons do, when flying in a commercial plane.

GRATEFUL GIFTS

A patient's gratitude and their parents' appreciation is the best reward a surgeon can receive, touching their heart, motivating, inspiring and giving strength to continue practicing their beautiful profession. A patient's parents are extremely grateful for a doctor's work and want to present them with what they think is something very good, something they would enjoy. I have a long list of stories related to the kind of gifts that people gave to me over the years.

I remember a child from my private practice in Mexico that I operated on successfully. His father came to the office for a post operative visit and explained that he had no money to pay; he asked if I could wait for him to pay. I told him not to worry about it. The next day, the father came back and walked into my office. "Dr. Peña, I have not been able to get the money to pay for the operation, but I have decided to give you something that I value very much." He put something on my desk and quickly left my office.

When I looked in the package, I found the medal that he won during a swimming competition at the Pan American Games representing Mexico! I thought that it was unacceptable for me to receive that present, so I took the medal and ran out looking for the young man but I could not find him. In fact, he never came back.

During my practice in Mexico City, I had the opportunity to operate on the child of a painter; an excellent artist named Jorge Flores. Like most artists at the beginning of their careers, he was struggling to provide the basic needs for his wife and three children. His son required a simple, one-hour operation that was performed uneventfully. One week later, during the post-operative visit, Jorge asked me if I could wait a few months to receive my payment. My answer was, "Don't worry about it. Forget it."

A month went by and unexpectedly Jorge showed up at my house with a beautiful, very large painting—a gift for me. I was overwhelmed and explained to him that the cost of that piece of art probably would be equivalent to the price of 15 of the operations that I had performed on his son. To that, Jorge replied, "Dr. Peña, for an operation like the one you performed on my son, I could make 15 paintings like this one."

*****

During one of my busy clinic days at INP, a family from a little town in the mountains inquired if I liked animals. I answered that I like them very much. The next week I got a call from hospital security that there was a family with a full grown goat that they brought for me. I explained to the family that even though I like goats, I could not accept that particular present because a live animal was not allowed in the hospital. The family showed a little disappointment and decided to go back home.

The following week they showed up at the clinic with a big sack. They had killed the goat and brought all the fresh portions of meat and bones to me as a gift. They said that cooking this animal was delicious and I should try it at home. Actually, I did not have a particular interest in eating goat but I did not want to be rude to the grateful parents, so I accepted their offering. I was in the middle of a busy clinic and the question was what to do with the plastic bag of fresh goat meat. I walked around the floor, found a big refrigerator and decided to put the bag inside. I went back to the clinic and continued working. At the end of the day, I was tired and forgot all about the big sack. I went home for the weekend.

The next Monday, I arrived at the hospital and when I entered my office I found a big turmoil. My secretary was agitated and there were two head nurses speaking with her. The police were called to investigate the body of a child cut into pieces that was found in a plastic bag in one of the refrigerators! I was alarmed and could not believe what I was hearing. Suddenly, I remembered the goat. I was extremely embarrassed. I explained everything and called the police to tell them not to come. As compensation for such grief, I distributed the goat meat amongst everybody that was interested.

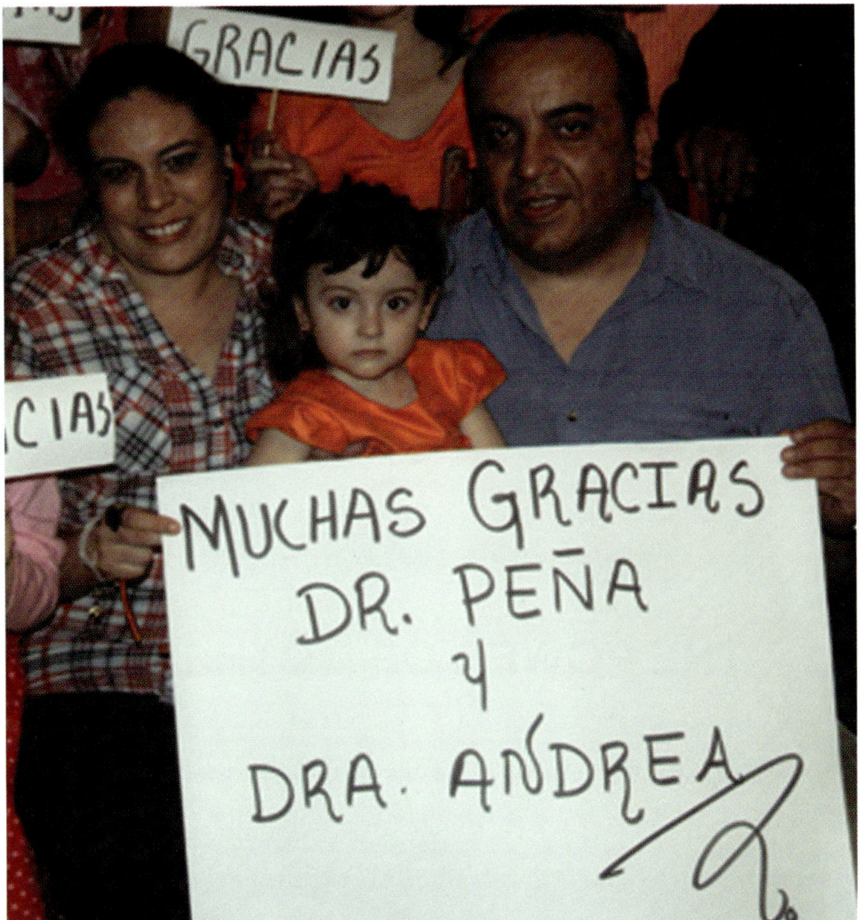

Mariá José

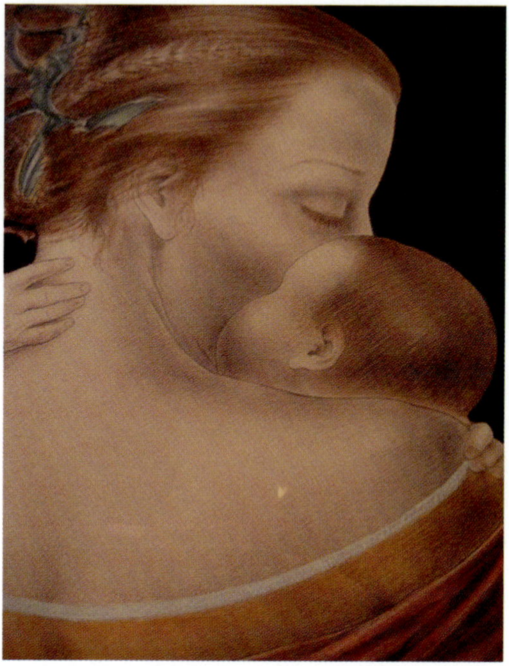

THE POWER OF MOTHERS

A child born with a serious congenital malformation represents a devastating and serious challenge for parents. It occurs randomly and unannounced, having a dramatic impact on a family's life. This is particularly tragic when the malformation produces significant sequelae, handicapping the patient for life.

An old person in poor health is certainly something sad, but somehow, understanding life and the temporary nature of human existence helps to accept disease and death in the elderly. On the contrary, serious congenital malformations, chronic diseases and the death of a child are nearly impossible to accept. Deep inside, regardless of religious or philosophical convictions, there is something intrinsically wrong when a very abnormal, painful event is inflicted upon a young innocent creature.

Observing parents' multiple reactions is a painful and magnificent lesson in human nature. Babies with severe defects may be born into a privileged environment, becoming part of a family of educated people with means enough to care for them. The arrival of the child with such maladies, making him a patient for life, jolts the couple that thought everything could be planned and done successfully. In this kind of environment, the family is shocked—in spite of all the resources and possibilities, there is a limit to what they can do for their child. A similar situation may occur to a very humble couple with six children or in a family with an alcoholic father, living under very precarious circumstances. I have seen couples divorce. I have seen fathers leave and never come back. I also met good fathers who react in a positive way, contributing significantly to the welfare of the ailing child and the family. In general, though, mothers represent the most powerful element in the stability of the family and the benefit of their sick child. Mothers are the ones who remain close to the child and struggle limitlessly.

During my 14 years of practicing pediatric surgery in Mexico, I was exposed to two totally distinct worlds: the world of the private practice and the world of the public health hospital. The private practice was comprised of middle class, high middle class and wealthy people, with resources to pay for the best medical and surgical care, whereas the public health hospital saw children of extremely poor families, with no insurance and no resources. Impressively, the sensitivity, solidarity, compliance and dedication of mothers were very similar in both of these groups.

Some of my colleagues in Mexico used to say that it was very complicated to conduct long-term assessments in public hospitals because patients were not compliant and they did not make it to their appointments. I cannot disagree with them more; my experience was quite different. My patients met their appointments most of the time. It was remarkable to see mothers and their children travel hundreds of miles to spend the night before a consultation on the hospital sidewalk, just to be on time for an appointment. Some of those same mothers are still in contact with me, sharing what has happened to their children now that they are adults. I have a great deal of admiration and respect for them.

After my years of practice in Mexico, I was invited to occupy a significant position as chief of surgery of a children's hospital in New York. Since I was very successful in Mexico, both academically and in private practice, it took me a long time to decide to leave my country. Friends explained that a big reason for my success in Mexico was because I was Mexican—I knew the idiosyncrasies of my patients and their parents and I related very well with them. I understood their sense of humor, their cultural background and their religion. Moving to another country, speaking another language, having much less knowledge of the culture and ideology could represent a major obstacle in becoming equally successful. I had serious concerns about this but finally decided to make the move.

Now, 25 years later, I have learned much more than I had expected and I do not regret my decision. I have been equally successful, if not more so, in this country. The United States is a multicultural country and one cannot make generalizations about the characteristics of American mothers. Not only have I interacted with American mothers but I also interacted with mothers from all over the world (thanks to my travels). What impressed me most is that the dedication, passion and strength to fight for their children are universal traits of all mothers. Mothers, everywhere, also have the capacity and sensitivity to detect doctors who are sincerely and authentically interested in their children.

MARTHA

While in New York, I received a letter from Martha, a mother of a child from a poor South American country. She explained that her child was born with Hirschsprung's disease[88] and had an operation in one of the government hospitals. The operation failed—her child had severe complications and nearly died. He was left with a colostomy[89] and the doctors told her that they had reached the

88 Condition in which part of the baby's colon does not have adequate nerves resulting in a lack of necessary propulsive movement of the bowel.

89 Opening from the colon through the abdominal wall to the outside of the body for excretion.

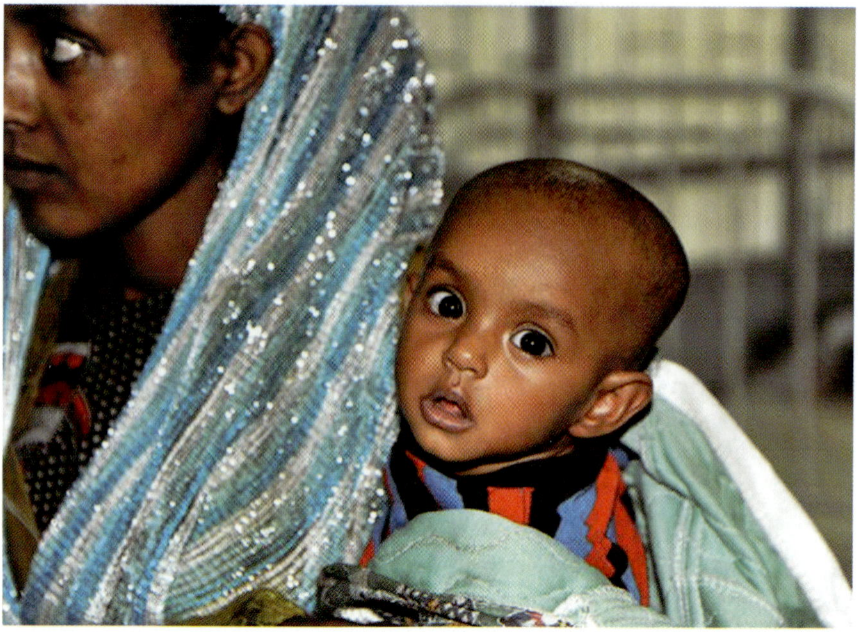

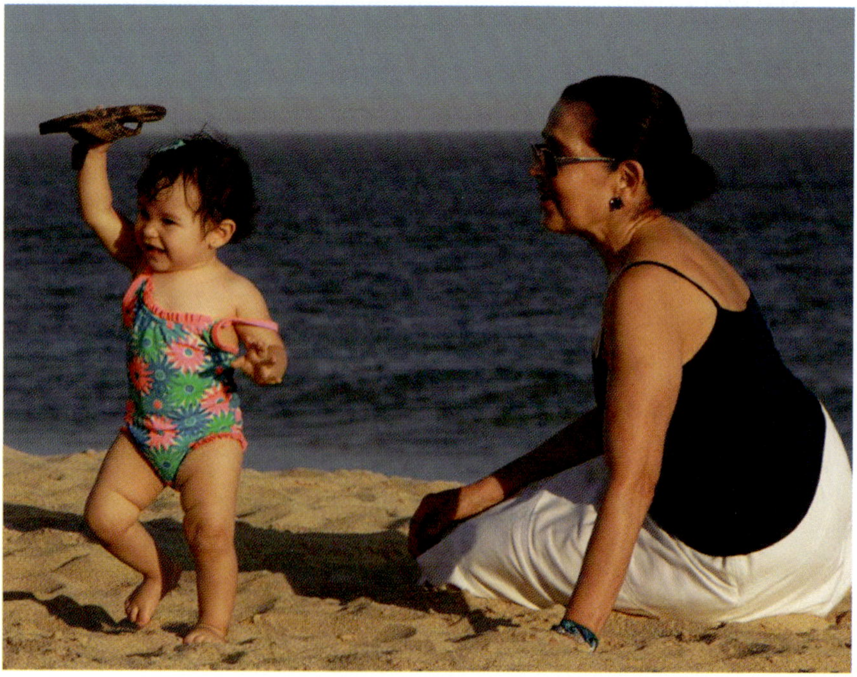

limit of what they could do for him. Like most mothers, she was not intimidated and did not accept that as an end. Being poor and uneducated did not stop her from finding other possibilities to improve her son's condition. Here, common sense lead her to believe that a government institution provoked the damage in her son, so it was the government's obligation to pay for the repair. She wrote a letter to me. I requested some x-rays and her son's medical records, which were sent to me. She revealed that she requested her government to pay for her trip to New York as well as the re-operation of her son. I did not want to disappoint her, so I did not tell her that I thought she would be facing an impossible task and that they would never come to New York.

Martha went to the hospital and explained what she wanted to the director. The director claimed there was nothing he could do and discouraged her from trying to get funds from the government to take her son to the United States. She was not dispirited and moved, systematically, through the numerous levels of bureaucracy of her country's health system. About a year later, at last, Martha reached the office of the secretary of health. Of course, she was told that the secretary could not see her, to which the mother replied that she would wait until he could. They explained to her that she did not have an appointment and she answered that she wanted to arrange one. They said there were no appointments available and she explained that she would wait until there was one. She decided not to leave the office and many days later, an exasperated secretary of health decided to see her.

Soon after the meeting, Martha sent me a letter saying that she had obtained the necessary resources from the government to come to the United States. I operated on her son in New York and fortunately, I was able to restore his anatomy and function. Perhaps, for someone with the pleasure of living in a rich, developed country, this story does not mean much; however, traveling or living abroad, allows one to appreciate more of the merit of this mother.

NATASHA

When the Soviet Union and the United States had very little communication due to the Cold War, a little baby was born in Russia with an anorectal malformation. The child received only a temporary colostomy. Natasha, the mother, decided that her child would benefit from receiving the main repair of the malformation in New York. The decision was a little problematic because the United States did not grant visas to Russian citizens and the Soviet government did not allow Russians to go to the United States. Natasha, however, was able to gain a visa to Italy and remained there for one entire year, trying to find a way to travel to the United States. Eventually, she made it and I had the privilege of meeting both mother and baby. Her child had a malformation with a favorable prognosis and the result of the operation was very good. When I operated on this patient, Natasha could not speak English.

During the following weeks she studied English and six months later, she was fluent. She never returned to Russia. Eventually, Natasha decided to go to nursing school and became a very efficient nurse at our own institution.

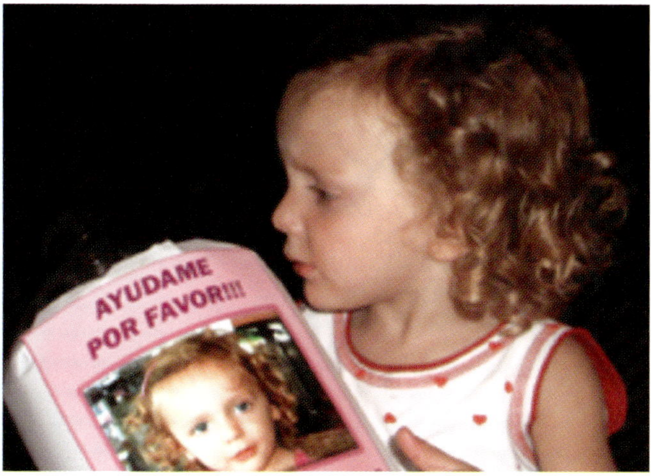

TODO POR PAULINA

A few months ago, I received an email from a desperate mother from a South American country. She explained that her daughter, Paulina, was born with a complex anorectal and urogenital malformation. Paulina had an attempted failed repair and had a colostomy. The mother had read about the Colorectal Center at Cincinnati Children's Hospital on the Internet and requested help for her daughter. The email was so moving that I decided to contact her, which was not an easy task. I had to phone one of her relatives who lived close to her so we could talk. She asked how much the operation would cost in the United States. Feeling sorry and almost embarrassed, I gave her an estimate. The cost of medicine in the United States, in terms of the local currency in most countries of the world, is exorbitant and the cost of an operation like the one Paulina required may represent the total salary of an entire lower middle class family for ten years or even more.

When she realized that it was almost impossible for her daughter to be operated on in the US she asked if there was any possibility that I could travel to her country to operate. I explained that I required an invitation from the local surgeons plus the legal authorization from the health authorities for my wife, Dr. Andrea Bischoff (also a pediatric surgeon), and I to operate in her country. We would do the operation for free but she would have to find the resources to pay the local hospital, as well as our traveling expenses. She said she would contact me soon.

Two months later, I got a phone call from the mother saying that everything was ready. She got enough money to pay for our trip, the hospital, anesthesiologist and assistants. She made all of the necessary bureaucratic arrangements for us to operate on Paulina in her country and she convinced the local pediatric surgeons to extend us an invitation. We were authorized to operate in her country and she obtained privileges for us occupy the best private hospital of the city.

When we arrived, we found that everybody, from the people in the airport to the people in the street, knew about this lower middle class mother. She started a campaign to raise funds: "Todo por Paulina" ("Everything for Paulina") included raffles, dance parties and races. Paulina's family and friends even sold bottles of water to car drivers waiting at traffic lights. Very soon, the power of this mother and solidarity of the community raised the necessary funds! Andrea and I had the privilege to repair the defect and we also organized a short course on the surgical treatment of anorectal malformations for the local pediatric surgeons.

LA JAROCHA

When I was an intern at the Central Military Hospital in Mexico, I took care of the son of a sergeant. His mother, an uneducated poor lady, was extremely compliant, dedicated, sensitive and loving. She was always alert to the baby's needs. The mother was particularly sociable, making friends with all of the nurses and other mothers in the ward. She came from the coast of the Gulf of Mexico so everybody knew her by the name of La Jarocha—a non-pejorative term used to designate people from that part of the country. She liked to be called by that name. The baby had a chronic condition and required frequent venous access. Due to his condition, his veins were not easy to find. I was persistent and lucky to find his veins, something the mother appreciated very much. I developed a special rapport with the child and his mother.

At that time, I was doing a rotation internship and could only spend one month in each department. After only one month, when I left the pediatric department to continue my rotation, I was called because La Jarocha demanded my presence. The chief of pediatrics, also a colonel, explained that the mother complained to him because she was not happy with the care her child was receiving. The colonel specifically designated a third year resident to care for her baby but she was still unhappy. The colonel offered to assign a fully trained attending pediatrician for her child but she refused. Finally, the colonel offered to personally care for her son but La Jarocha declined—she wanted me to take care of her son. Even though I was only a first year intern and no longer part of the pediatric team, the chief was so exasperated that he paged me to go and care for her child. I felt extremely honored by such a request.

The sergeant, the mother and I developed a very special relationship. She used to call me at home for every problem her child had. That went on for several years during my surgical and pediatric training in Mexico. Eventually, the time came for me to move to the United States to continue my training in Boston. While living in Boston for those three years, I was never able to go to Mexico due to economical limitations (characteristic of a surgeon in training). When I finally returned to Mexico, on the very day that I showed up to work at the Central Military Hospital, waiting for me at the entrance was La Jarocha with her child! She had found out when I was returning. She knew where I would be and wanted me to continue caring for her child.

*****

During one of the frequent admissions, La Jarocha had a conversation (as usual) with a mother of another child who was in the next bed. The mother was crying and said that her child had leukemia and he was very sick. Her child needed a special type of chemotherapy but the hospital did not have the specific drug for the treatment. They were waiting for the hospital administration to buy the medicine. One week had already passed and the administration failed to do so; her child was getting worse. La Jarocha, full of enthusiasm, pleaded the mother not to worry. La Jarocha would take care of it.

She grabbed the mother by the arm and they both walked out of the hospital and took a taxi to the main radio station in Mexico City. On-air, La Jarocha explained the mother's predicament. Within a few hours, millions of Mexicans knew that at the Central Military Hospital in Mexico City, there was a very sick child who desperately needed a medication to save his life and the hospital was not able to buy it. The radio station requested donations to help the child. La Jarocha and the mother were extremely happy. They took a taxi back to the hospital, knowing that something good was going to happen.

At the entrance of the hospital, several military police soldiers were waiting for them. It seemed it was unacceptable to advertise that the Central Military Hospital was not buying a drug for a leukemic child who was also the son of a soldier. The military police took these two ladies directly to the office of the major general director. The general was extremely upset—this could be a very serious problem and he could lose his job. He screamed at the ladies. The mother of the sick child was sobbing and extremely afraid. La Jarocha, though, did not look intimidated. She patiently waited until the general finished his vociferating speech, full of threats and admonitions. Then she spoke.

"Listen, Sir, you are a general. My husband is only a sergeant. So, you can scream and give orders to him. I am humble and poor but I am not in the military. You cannot scream at me and you cannot give me orders. As soon as I leave this room, I am going back to the radio station *and* to the newspapers to tell everybody what you just told us!"

The general paled, contained his anger and ordered his assistant to buy the medication immediately. He then respectfully asked the ladies to leave his office. La Jarocha and her friend were very pleased and went back to the floor to be near the sick child.

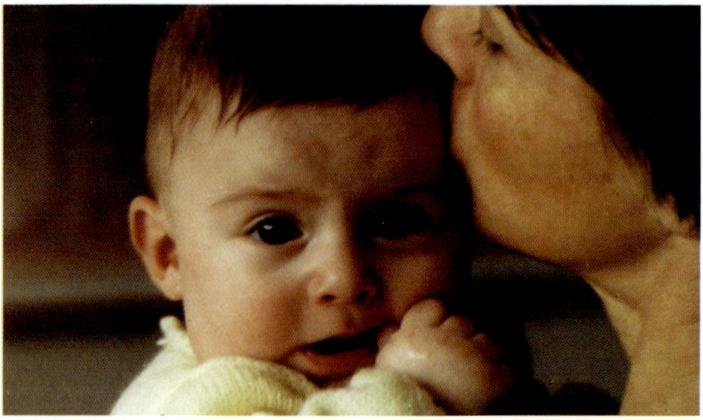

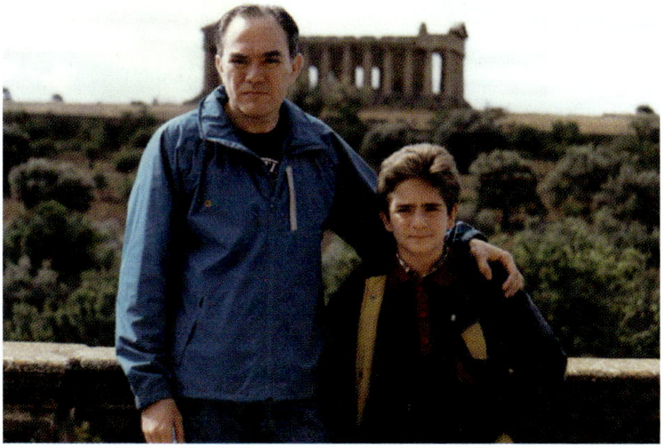

SICILIAN MIGHT

Many years ago, I had the honor of traveling to Italy to operate on a child from Sicily. The parents, as usual, were very grateful and extended a generous invitation to visit them in Agrigento, Sicily (famous for its beautiful Roman ruins, receiving visitors from all over the world). The family, like most Sicilian families, was extremely warm, friendly and generous.

Arriving in Agrigento, I was happily surprised to find that I would be staying at the most luxurious hotel in the city. Not only that, but I was in the Presidential Suite which had a very wide terrace located strategically in front of the most famous Roman building in the ruins. At night, one could open the window and contemplate the illuminated remains from bed.

The morning after my first night in that beautiful place, a group of British tourists stopped me upon returning from breakfast. "Excuse us, Sir. Are you staying in that particular room?" I told them

I was. "Well, you are very privileged. We specifically requested that room and it was impossible to get. We're from England. We heard about that room because when Queen Elizabeth visited Agrigento, she stayed there." I was very surprised by their information and then they asked, "What did you have to do to get that room?"

My answer was very simple, "I operated on a child." With that, I went to my beautiful suite feeling very proud of my work.

After touring the beautiful ruins, while driving to my friends' house, I was curious and asked my patient's father, "How did you manage to get that luxurious suite for me? I heard from some British tourists that it is extremely hard to get."

He smiled, "Actually, it was very easy, Dr. Peña. You see, I work for the city's telephone company. I went to the manager of the hotel and said, 'I want the Presidential Suite for Dr. Peña. If you don't give me the room, you will have no phone service for one week.'"

DOLORES

During my time as INP director, I decided to make myself available to anybody who wanted to talk to me. Accordingly, I instructed my secretary to allow everybody to meet me as soon as possible. I wanted to hear firsthand the complaints from our patients' parents. That strategy allowed me to learn many important lessons; I also lived many interesting episodes during this time.

One morning, my secretary told me about the mother of an outpatient who wanted to see me. She walked into my office with another female relative who called her Dolores. Her name was Dolores Gonzalez. She carried a child in her arms, covered with her shawl. Dolores was poor. She had three children and her husband worked in a factory making a meager salary that was barely enough to survive. She wanted to see me because the doctors in the hospital told her that her son needed, as soon as possible, an operation called fundoplication[90] to avoid aspiration pneumonias[91] and the possibility of death. With some hesitation, she agreed to the operation. When Dolores learned that the operation had to be done six months later due to an excessive workload in the operating room, she became very disappointed. Her common sense allowed her to perceive a great inconsistency—and she made a formal complaint to me. I listened to her until she calmed down, then I asked some questions.

"Mrs. Gonzalez, how old is your son?"

"Six years old," she replied.

"Where is he?"

"Right here," she said, uncovering the child in her arms.

I was shocked to see that she was carrying her six-year-old child in her arms. Very soon into our discussion, I found the explanation for her son's problems—the child suffered from severe brain damage consecutive to a complicated delivery. He was constantly drooling, his eyes and body moved in a non-coordinated way, his weight

90 Surgical procedure designed to avoid gastroesophageal reflux, which is the abnormal regurgitation of food from the stomach into the esophagus.

91 Inflammation of the lungs caused by inhaling or choking on vomit.

was equivalent to that of a two-year-old child and he wore diapers, he did not respond to his name and could not articulate a word. I then scoured through the child's voluminous medical records and found that Dolores had been faithfully and consistently bringing her child to the hospital for six years. She had weekly visits to the rehabilitation department, plus multiple visits to the ER for episodes of pneumonia, urinary tract infections and other related disorders. She never missed an appointment in spite of the fact that she lived far away and it took her two hours to travel from her house to the hospital with public transportation. The child underwent several orthopedic operations to correct contractures and deformities. Dolores was a very responsible, concerned, dedicated mother and managed to take care of this sick child in addition to all of her other family responsibilities.

She continued explaining her concerns. "I want the best for my child. I want him to be like the others."

Then, I dared to ask Mrs. Gonzalez what she expected for her son in the future.

"The doctors told me that if I continue with the rehabilitation, my son will improve."

"And how much improvement do you expect?"

"I expect him to be like all the other children, to go to school and be happy."

"Mrs. Gonzalez, I am sorry but I must be honest with you. Your son will never be 'normal.' The operation may avoid aspiration pneumonias but it is not going to improve or cure his brain damage. I will be happy to help you to get an earlier date for the operation if that is what you want. But it is very important for you to know what to expect."

Dolores remained silent for a couple of minutes then, with tears in her eyes, she replied, "How come nobody told me that before? If I had known that six years ago, I would have been at home with my son." Dolores expressed her appreciation, hugged me and left my office weeping. She never came back.

I still wonder how many mothers in the world are living through this same sad saga and just how thorough the information from their doctors really is.

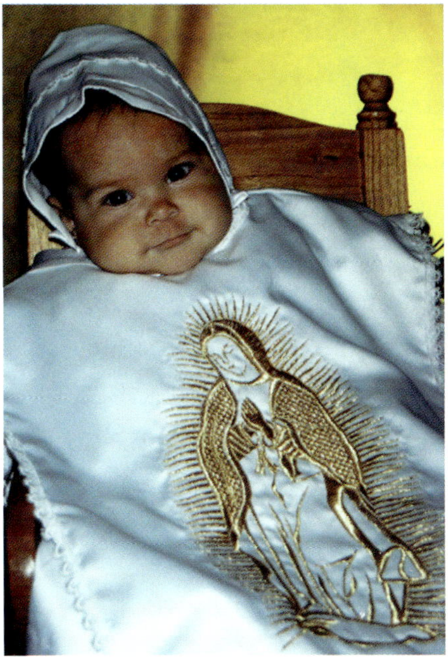

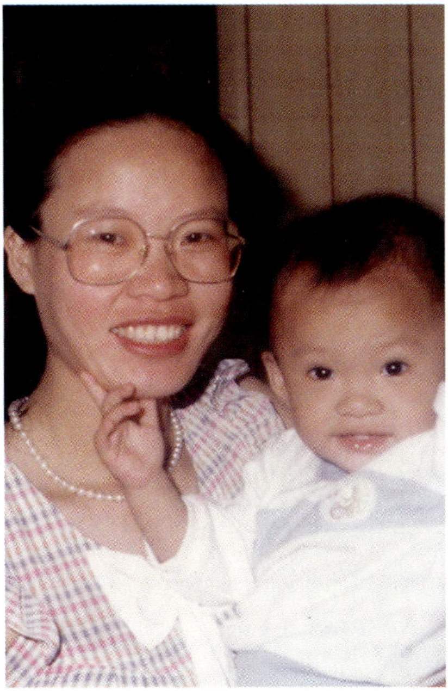

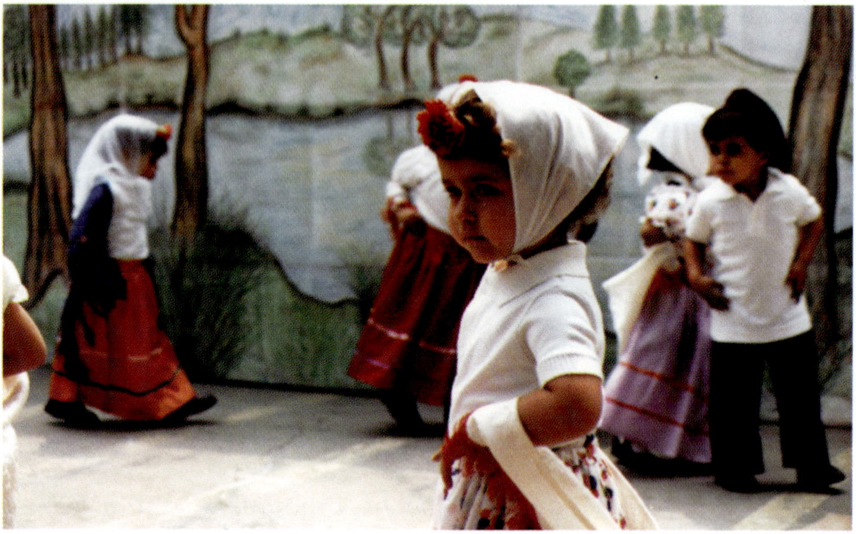

THE POWER OF CHILDREN

Children are ingenious, sincere, naïve, creative, spontaneous and charming: all the qualities humans tend to shed as they grow older. While working with children, doctors are transported into a magical realm, never having to step foot outside the work place. Sometimes, while making rounds, a doctor is upset about some problems of his daily routine. Then, the doctor visits with a sick child who says something enchanting and powerful, impacting his mood. He cannot avoid laughing, realizing the enormous privilege of dealing with such a sweet, innocent soul.

ANNIE

While writing this particular paragraph, I interrupted my

progress because it was getting late and I still had to make rounds. As usual, I was in a hurry with many things passing through my mind. Among my in-patients was Annie, a lovely 2½-year-old girl that I had operated on a few days earlier. The nurses and a resident joined me to visit the patients. When we entered Annie's room, she was sitting in her mother's lap, carefully holding her doll in her arms in a sweet, maternal manner. I said hello to everybody and asked how Annie was doing. There was no answer; then I looked at Annie and found that she had her right index finger on her mouth and nose, indicating that I should lower my voice because her doll was trying to fall asleep. The rest of the visit in Annie's room was carried out in a whisper. After this visit, I went to see my other patients feeling reinvigorated and happy.

LUCHO

Working in Mexico at INP, I was busy making rounds surrounded by all of the residents of my team, as well as the nurses of the surgical floor. While standing beside, we would discuss the diagnosis, the operation conducted the night before, vital signs, laboratory results and what should be the next step in the management of the patient. I vividly remember one particular child, approximately six years old, who came from the coast of Mexico. His name was Lucho. He was a very poor child. The residents told me that he had undergone an exploratory laparotomy[92] due to a bowel perforation.[93] During those years in Mexico, it was very common to see poor children with intestinal perforations due to salmonella or amoeba.[94] Lucho was receiving intravenous fluids, had a tube running through his nose into the stomach and a catheter in his bladder.

While discussing his case, Lucho was listening carefully. Obviously, he could not understand anything about medicine but his eyes were wide, showing a great deal of interest. At the end of the discussion, we concluded about the amount of intravenous fluids that Lucho would receive, the antibiotics that would be best for him and a potential prognosis. We decided to move to the next patient.

"Pssst."

Lucho was calling me, moving his index finger. He wanted me to get close to him. I sat on the bed and leaned over, placing my ear close to his face. He wanted to tell me something but did not want anyone else to hear. When I was close enough, he whispered, "You're the chief, right?"

"Yes, I am."

He said, "If you tell the nurses to feed me, I will give you some money."

Lucho was extremely poor and did not have any money. He was very hungry. He had learned that in his young life, in order to

---

92 Incision through the abdominal wall.

93 Abnormal opening in a hollow organ made by a rupture or injury.

94 A bacteria and a parasite, respectively, that are very commonly seen in poor countries.

survive in his town, he had to be very clever. He learned to bribe! During the conversation with the residents and nurses, he had been watching carefully. He was trying to determine whom the key person was to contact so that he could eat. He thought that he was not getting food because he was not bribing somebody. Supported by his survival instinct, Lucho used his intuition and detected me as the head of the group. Lucho decided to go straight to the top, adhering to a traditional Mexican principle:

To solve a problem, talk to God, not to angels.

I felt like laughing and crying at the same time.

LITTLE ARABIC GIRL

Many years later, working in New York, I received the medical records of a little girl suffering from a complex urogenital and colorectal malformation. The medical records came from an Arabic country. The government authority of that country requested my evaluation, diagnosis and management plan. After I elaborated all of that, the government decided to send the girl to New York so I could operate on her, paying all of the expenses. We fixed a specific date for the operation. Two days before, I received a phone call from the country's embassy in Washington D. C. "Dr. Peña, we wanted to notify you that your patient is already here in Washington and is ready to travel to New York for the operation. But there seems to be a problem. We have found out that you work in a Jewish hospital. This embassy cannot make a check for any kind of Jewish organization."

There was silence on the line and then I spoke, "Well, I am very sorry, because the only one who will suffer under these circumstances is this little girl."

Silence again. Then the man asked, "Dr. Peña, is there any other way to take care of this problem?"

Déjà vu! I had heard that in my past life. In Mexico, we used that phrase when we wanted to solve a problem using ingenious, non-orthodox paths (like bribing). "Yes, there is a way. Your organization cannot make checks to a Jewish institution and I work for a Jewish institution *but* I am not Jewish. Your embassy could make a check for me and I will make a check for the Jewish organization. What about that?"

An enthusiastic voice spoke up on the other side of the phone, "Dr. Peña, that was exactly what I had in mind but I did not know if you would accept something like that."

"It would be my pleasure."

The official from that embassy was brave enough to find a way to go around the rules of his embassy and I found a way to go around the rules of my hospital. The hospital was paid, I operated on the girl, the operation was highly successful and the family was very happy! This incident illustrates the power of a little girl but in addition, is an example of the universal character of surgery and medicine. When looking at patients, physicians do not recognize political nor territorial boundaries. They do not perceive the color of the skin, religion, nor political orientation.

ANNA

On a routine clinic day, I met for the first time a very pretty Chinese girl and her father, Craig, an educated American man. For one week, Kathie Guardino (my dedicated and inspired nurse with whom I have worked closely with for over 15 years) and I implemented our Bowel Management Program for Anna. This program aimed to maintain cleanliness in children with disorders in bowel control.

Kathie and I were surprised that Anna's father personally helped to implement our program. Typically, it was the mother who dealt with such issues. He was reliable, committed and consistent—all the attributes required to be successful with this kind of management. The devotion and loving care that this man provided to his child was remarkable

While I was giving the final recommendations during their last visit, I prodded a bit and dared to ask Craig when their plane was leaving. Craig replied that the plane would leave whenever he decided. It impressed me how this man, obviously very wealthy and influential, was so dedicated and personally involved in caring for this adopted girl. This is when I learned about their story.

Craig was a prominent American businessman and he decided to retire early due to health-related problems. As an inspired, sensitive human being, he traveled to China and visited an orphanage. While walking through the house, one of the orphans, a little nine-month-old girl, stared at him from the moment he entered the room. He came close to her and she grabbed his index finger and decided not to let go while the man talked to the managers. This touched the man's heart and he decided to adopt the girl.

Craig is one of those rare fathers who actually gives primary care to his child. He is an extremely meticulous and sensitive human being. I have been watching this little girl grow and have perceived how intelligent, charismatic and beautiful of an American girl she has become. I cannot help but wonder who was the lucky person in this inspiring relationship? The little girl born in China, left in an orphanage and adopted by a wealthy, generous American who can make her dreams come true and give her a wonderful future? Or the proud father whom now has brightness in his eyes and enjoys having such a wonderful girl as his daughter? Anna is becoming a talented and sweet girl, growing up, surrounded by love. An inspired father, Craig has used his resources and valuable time to benefit thousands of children as a president of a board of trustees of a very important American children's hospital.

Since then, the Colorectal Center for Children at Cincinnati Children's Hospital has operated on over 100 Chinese girls born with an anorectal malformation and adopted by American parents. It is very impressive to see so many philanthropic Americans adopt

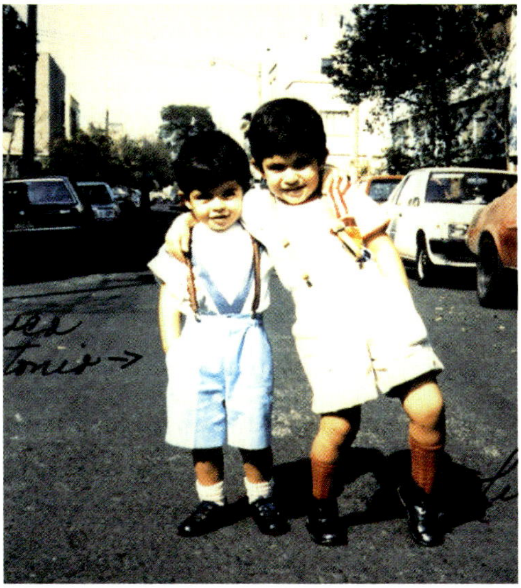

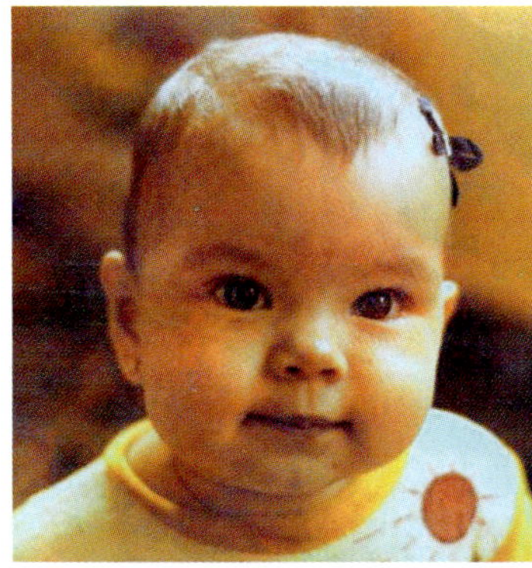

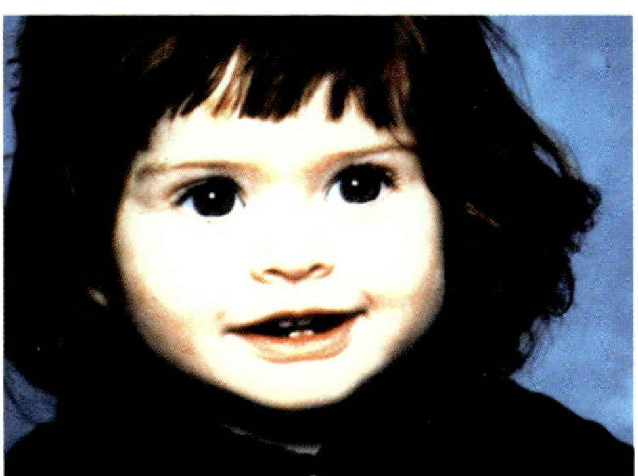

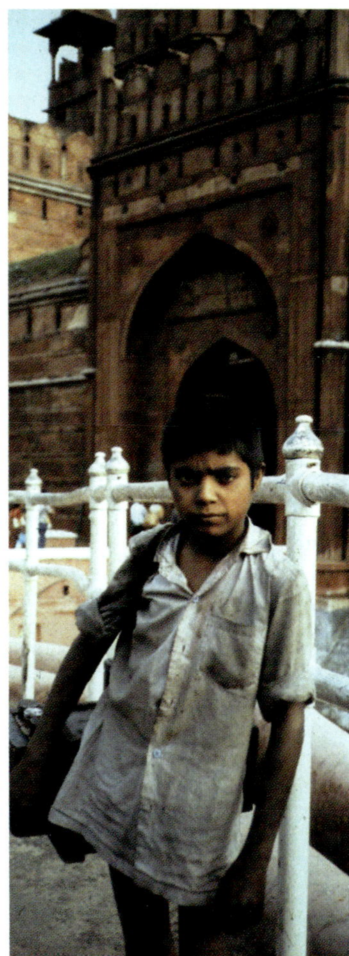

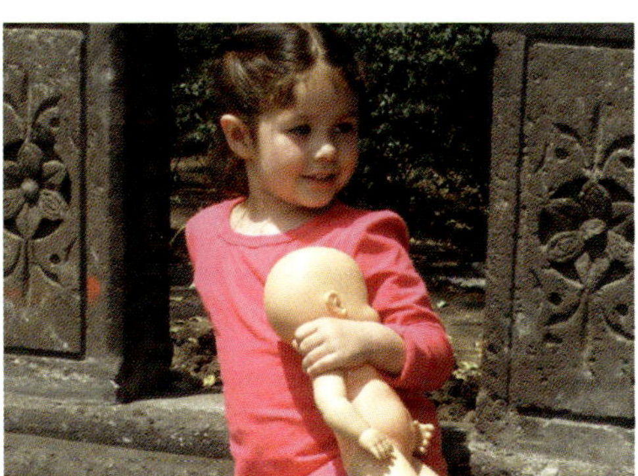

children with health problems because they know they can help them.

SAMSON

In the spring of 1974, during one of my clinic days, I saw a patient by the name of Samson, referred by a doctor from a faraway place in Mexico. I was warned that Samson's mother was peculiar and had strange ideas. I consider these kinds of cases as personal challenges. I asked the nurse to bring the "peculiar mother" and her son to my cubicle. Samson turned out to be a very sociable, intelligent four-year-old and the mother seemed to be a nice lady. She explained that she had seen many doctors about Samson's problem but she had the feeling that the doctors did not pay attention to the things she described and as a consequence, nothing had been done to cure her child's problem.

One day, Samson's kindergarten teacher called her because she noticed something unusual while her class was singing the national anthem. The teacher saw something abnormal in Samson's neck while he was singing. But when Samson's mother saw him, he looked perfectly normal. The teacher explained that the abnormality only appeared when he was singing the national anthem. Samson was such a lovely, obedient child that when the teacher asked him to sing, he immediately did so with great enthusiasm. The Mexican national anthem reads, "Mexicanos al grito de Guerra." *Guerra* means war and it reaches a very high note and requires effort from children to reach it. Samson started singing and when he reached that high note, a huge bulging mass appeared in his neck! The mother was very worried and took him to the pediatrician.

The pediatrician laughed about that, examined the child, ordered some x-rays and some blood tests, reassured the mother and told her to go home. From there, she went to the state capital and asked for a head and neck specialist to look at Samson. He examined him, ordered some contrast studies and found everything to be normal. She then requested another consultation in Mexico City and that was why she was sitting next to me.

I found Samson to be completely normal, clinically speaking. But following an old, time-proven tradition of "listening to the mothers of your patients," I decided to have him to sing the national anthem. Samson sang with great gusto and when he reached the high note of "Guerra," a huge bulging mass protruded above his clavicle.[95] It was really impressive—it looked like it was going to burst at any minute!

Little Samson had congenital dilatation[96] of the internal jugular vein, a rare condition that has been described in medical literature. Sometimes, the dilatation affects veins in the chest; fortunately, Samson belonged to the group of patients that only had a dilatation of the vein in the neck and it was easy to treat and cure. Listening to mothers is an art that doctors must cultivate and teach to students

95 Either of two slender bones that extend from the upper part of the breastbone (sternum) to the shoulder. Collarbone.

96 In this case, inborn enlargement of a vein.

and residents. The information obtained is integral and valuable for the diagnosis.

TLALOC

When I returned to Mexico from Boston, I accepted the job as chief of surgery at the INP. The general director of INP warned me to be careful when I worked because I was young and all my attending surgeons (most of them older than me) would be watching me with great curiosity. He advised not to operate but rather make rounds and simply observe for a few weeks before acting, making decisions and treating patients. I tried to follow his advice, which has never been easy for me. I made rounds for a few days but then I was called to the infectious disease department to see a patient, a little two-month-old baby by the name of Tlaloc.

The name Tlaloc comes from Aztec mythology. Tlaloc was the Aztec god of rain. When the Aztec's needed more water they prayed to Tlaloc, who would send water from the skies. Many years ago, a huge monolithic statue of Tlaloc was discovered about three hours away from Mexico City. The Mexican government decided to "rescue" the huge sculpture and transport it to the garden of the anthropology museum. It was a very ingenious, expensive and hard working job to move that enormous piece of stone. The day Tlaloc was moved, Mexico City experienced the heaviest rain that it had seen in many years, lasting for many days.

I went with my residents to see baby Tlaloc; they called us

because he was jaundiced and was a diagnostic problem. The doctors were trying to decide whether it was a medical or surgical problem. Tlaloc was in the Infectious Disease department because the initial admission diagnosis was hepatitis.[97] Once again, besides consulting all the laboratory data and clinical evolution in the hospital, I decided to listen to the mother's story.

She was a non-educated mother with strong common sense. She explained that when Tlaloc was about three weeks old, he suddenly started to vomit forcefully—everything he ate was expelled far from his little body. She took him to Acapulco to be seen by a surgeon that decided to operate on him. It was found the Tlaloc suffered from a condition known as pyloric stenosis.[98] The operation went on for about two hours and after the procedure the baby looked very distended in his abdomen. The surgeon explained that the abdominal distention would go away and Tlaloc would recover very well. However, Tlaloc continued to be very sick and very distended. By day seven after the operation, the mother found that the wound on the abdomen was completely open and the bowel was lying in the baby's blankets. The surgeons, very alarmed, rushed him back to the operating room and closed the wound with bigger stitches. They even decided to put a very strong bandage around his abdomen. The mother said that Tlaloc started to improve but she noticed that his skin and eyes looked yellow. The

97 Inflammation of the liver caused by infectious or toxic agents and characterized by jaundice, fever, liver enlargement and abdominal pain.

98 Partial obstruction of the stomach outlet.

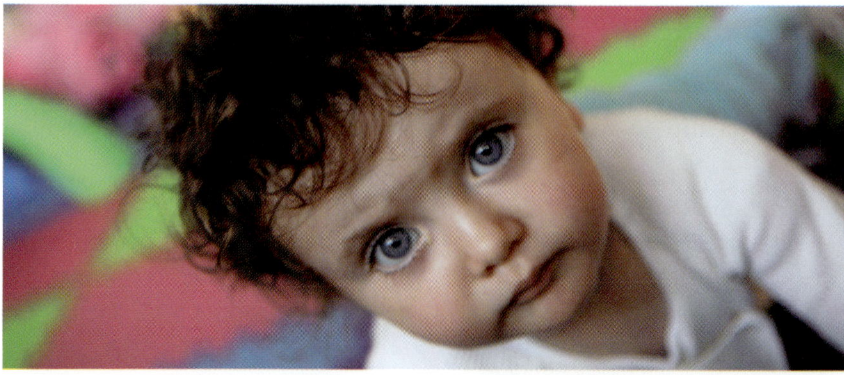

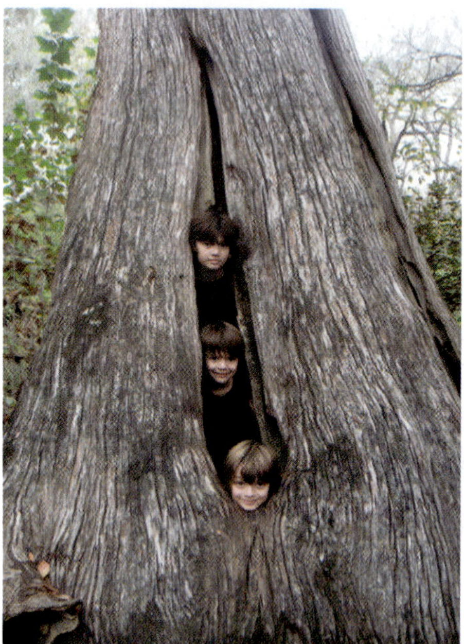

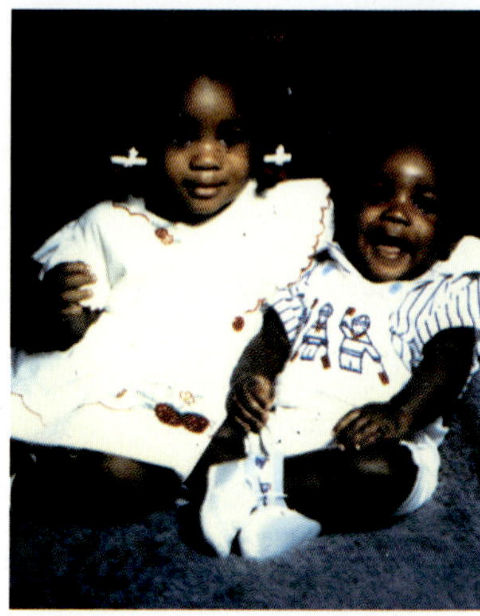

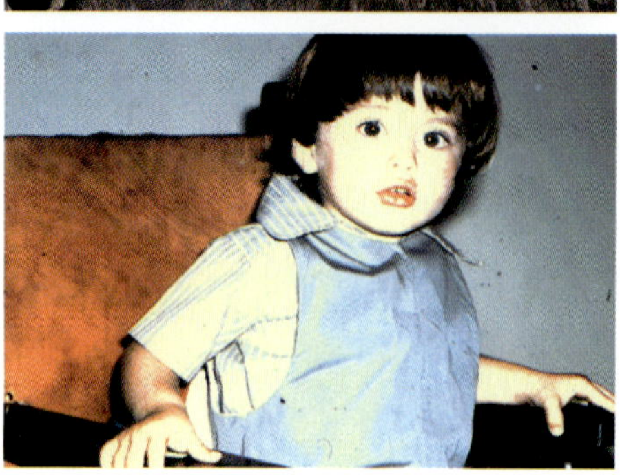

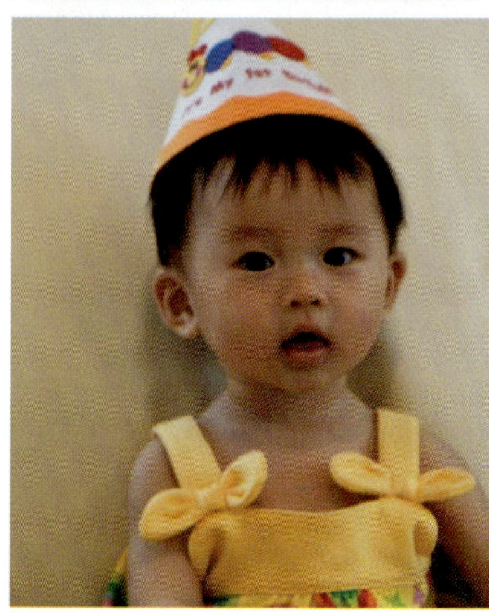

wound eventually healed but Tlaloc continued to have a distended abdomen and the yellowing was getting worse and worse.

The mother went from doctor to doctor and finally was referred to our institute. The laboratory tests, as I suspected, showed elevated direct bilirubin, indicating that he most likely had an obstruction of the bile ducts. Against the recommendation of the general director, I could not stand by any longer and I decided to take Tlaloc to the operating room that afternoon.

Because it was my first operation in this hospital, the operating room was filled with all the surgical residents and the surgical attendings. I suspected that they had a kind of morbid curiosity to see what kind of technical surgeon this 33 year old, new chief of surgery was. There are surgeons who do not accept observers in the operating room because they feel nervous; there are other surgeons who are indifferent about the presence of spectators, and of course, there is a third category (to which I confess I belong) with a big ego that enjoys very much to be surrounded by observers.

Tlaloc's mother was a humble uneducated lady yet she was able to describe a very consistent history with the clinical symptoms typical of pyloric stenosis—a condition usually cured with a 30-minute operation with typically excellent results. But when I surgically explored Tlaloc, as expected, I found that the bile ducts had been completely destroyed. When the surgeons tried to repair the pyloric stenosis, in some unexplained way, they tried to exteriorize[99] the pylorus[100] and literally tore apart the baby's bile ducts.

As a consequence of the rupture of the bile ducts, Tlaloc most likely had a lot of bile in the peritoneum[101], which provoked the abdominal distension and the dehiscence[102] of the abdominal suture and evisceration.[103] He managed to survive after all that! The bile ducts healed but he developed a biliary obstruction, manifested by severe jaundice. It was necessary to replace the bile ducts with a piece of his bowel and Tlaloc recovered uneventfully. Without fail, the day that I operated on Tlaloc, a big rainstorm started in Mexico City that lasted for three days.

SAMUEL

In the winter of 1974, I was called to see a newborn baby, underweight and premature; he was the son of a prominent wealthy family in Mexico City. He had obvious symptoms of intestinal obstruction. I operated on him and found that he had a condition called meconium peritonitis.[104] This is a bowel perforation that occurs when the baby is still in the mother's uterus. The intestinal obstruction is produced by heavily condensed or inspissated

99 To expose an internal organ or body part, as in surgery.

100 Ring of muscle that controls the passage of material from the stomach into the small intestine.

101 Transparent membrane lining the abdominal cavity that holds organs such as the intestines in place.

102 Separation of the layers of a surgical wound.

103 Disembowelment.

104 Refers to rupture of the bowel prior to birth, resulting in fetal stool (meconium) escaping in the surrounding space, leading to inflammation (peritonitis).

meconium[105] occurring as a part of a systemic disease known as cystic fibrosis.[106] I repaired the problem, reestablished the continuity of the bowel and put the baby in the newborn ICU.

These babies are not easy to manage because they frequently need ventilatory support. Babies with cystic fibrosis have problems due to the production of inspissated meconium but they also have respiratory problems due to condensed secretions in the airways. In those years in Mexico, the technology related to respiratory support, neonatal[107] intensive care and ventilators were not fully developed. The baby remained intubated for a long period of time and eventually I had to open a tracheostomy[108] to be able to better manage his airway. Samuel's bowel was working very well but his main trouble was now a respiratory one.

Two or three times per day I visited Samuel and answered hundreds of questions from his very anxious parents. In desperation, I told them that since they had the resources, they should take little Samuel to Children's Hospital Boston where the technology related with intensive care of these kinds of babies was much better than in Mexico City. The family did not hesitate and accepted my suggestion, instructing me to join them. I explained that I was a military doctor and could not leave the country without

105 First waste products to be discharged from the body in a newborn infant consisting of black mucus, bile and so forth.

106 Hereditary disease that mainly affects the lungs and digestive system, causing progressive disability and for some, early death.

107 Of or relating to the first 28 days of an infant's life.

108 Surgical construction of an opening in the trachea for the insertion of a catheter or tube to facilitate breathing.

special permission. The government did not give military people a passport without special consent from the secretary of defense. The father of the baby smiled, "Dr. Peña, you are coming with us. Tomorrow morning I will meet you at the government passport office. You will get your passport."

The next morning I was there and in about 15 minutes, because of the "special connections" of Samuel's parents, I got my official civilian passport—no questions asked. A private jet was rented to go to Boston. By removing some seats inside the plane, a special space was created to accommodate Samuel's transportation incubator[109] with batteries. I made a list of the material, equipment and medications that we required during the trip but we were unable to get a suction machine needed to frequently clean Samuel's tracheostomy tube. In order to suction the tracheostomy, I followed the most primitive technique, which is a suction done with a rubber bulb and a little catheter. I was ventilating the baby by hand, with a bag valve mask resuscitator because we had no respirator.

In the middle of the flight the incubator ran out of batteries. I took Samuel out and asked the pilot to increase the temperature of the cabin as high as possible. The baby's temperature was falling very rapidly and it was not easy to keep him warm. I decided to undress him and hold him near one of the plane's air vents, rotating his little body to expose him to the warm air. At times the mother helped me, holding him while I hand-ventilated him through the

109 Apparatus for maintaining optimal conditions (temperature, humidity, etc.) for growth and development, as one used in the early care of premature infants, or one used for cultures.

tracheostomy and suction the mucus from his airways. Everyone was sweating, very concerned because the baby looked more lethargic as time passed.

Finally, after several distressing hours, we arrived at the Boston airport where an ambulance was waiting. I went with the baby in the ambulance to the hospital. We put the baby in the ICU and connected him to the right type of ventilator. Samuel was very sick with respiratory alkalosis[110] produced by my over efficient hand ventilation. Once I felt the baby was safe, extremely exhausted, I went to sleep.

The following morning Samuel was doing much better. I went back to Mexico with my brand new civilian passport, allowing me to travel to many countries after that. Samuel stayed for about a month at the hospital but eventually died due to multiple respiratory complications. Samuel's family was very grateful in spite of the sad end of this story. They organized a special reception in Mexico City honoring doctors and nurses that tried to help little Samuel.

MANUELITO

By my last year of medical school, I had already decided that I liked children very much and therefore I showed a special interest and dedication to children. I tried to arrange things in such a way that I could spend more time than my classmates in the department of pediatrics. There, I met and treated a little child called Manuelito.

One day, I received a disheartening phone call from a family

110 Abnormally high alkalinity of the blood and body fluids.

member: my mother's sister, my aunt Esther, had attempted suicide and was taken to the Red Cross Hospital in Mexico City. I was asked if I could do anything for her. I was still not a graduated doctor but my family always came to me for advice whenever there was a medical problem. They were proud of me, they called me for every important medical decision and I was expected to advise them, even with the very poor knowledge of medicine that I had at that time. I suppose that happens in every family when they have a doctor as a member. They specifically wanted me to go to Aunt Esther and try to help her in some way. I decided to wear my white lab coat to look like a doctor and went to the Red Cross Hospital.

The Mexican Red Cross, for many years, has been a very important and revered institution in charge of responding to many emergencies in the giant Mexico City. Since the Mexican Red Cross was primarily supported by the generosity of the public it had many limitations. Red Cross ambulances were driven at very high speeds through the city and frequently involved in accidents, sometimes killing people rather than saving them. Inside the ambulances there was really nothing to help the patient with anyway. Still, everyone in Mexico loved the Red Cross because it was a non-profit organization manned mainly by volunteers, doing their best to help the injured and infirmed.

My aunt suffered from depression. She took an enormous amount of barbiturates and was found comatose in her bed. The Red Cross was notified and she was taken to their hospital.

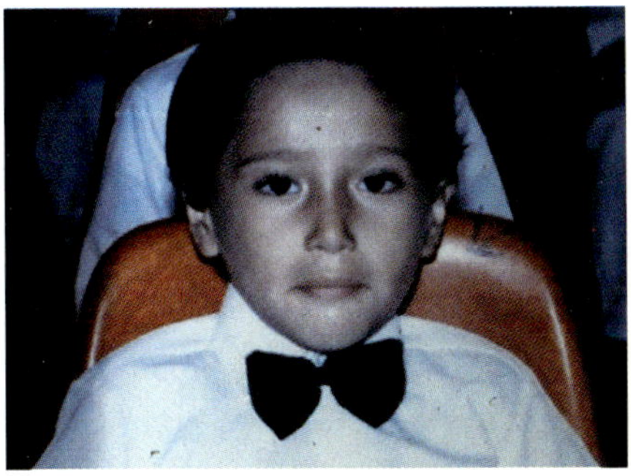

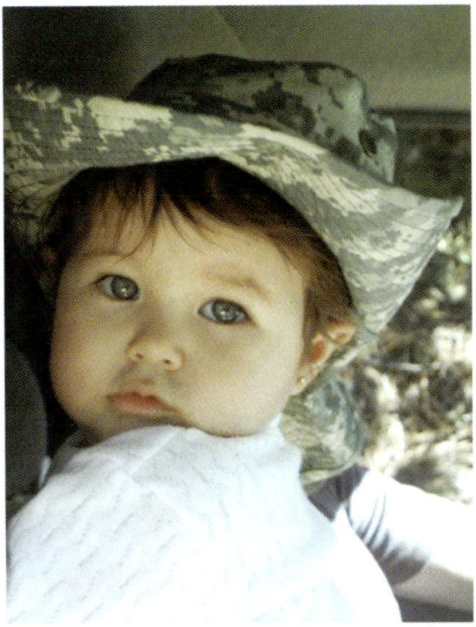

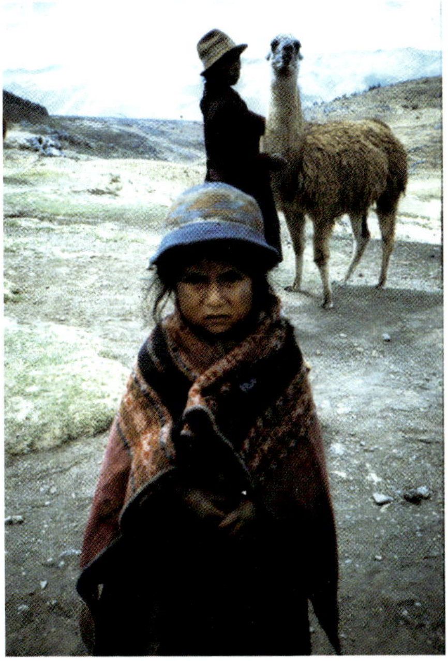

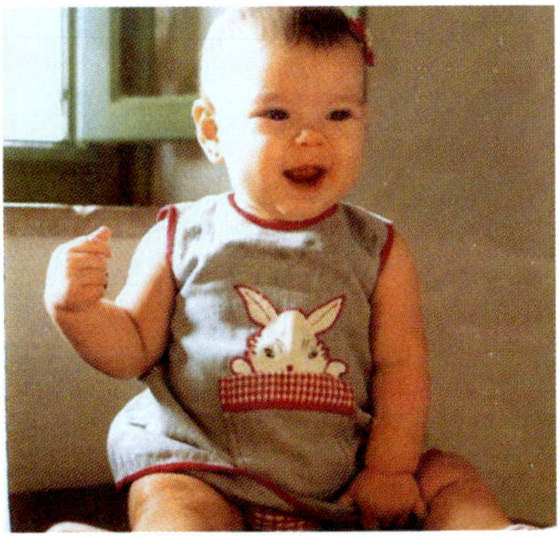

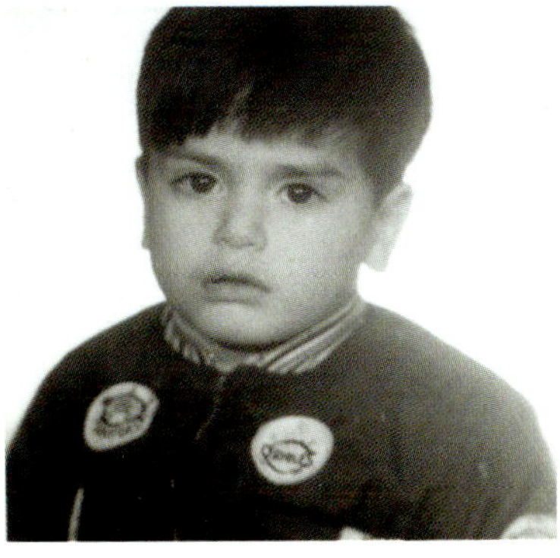

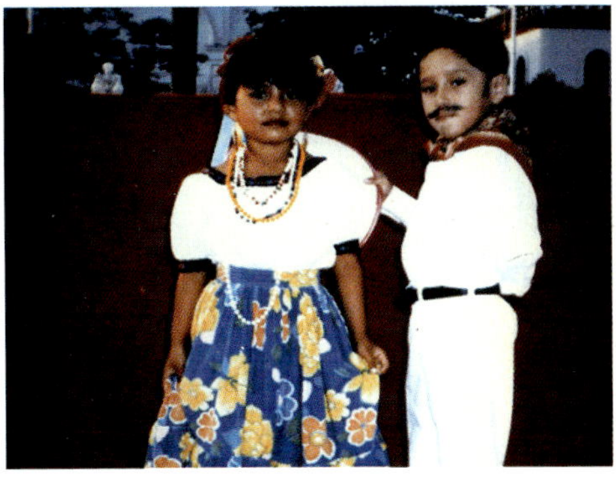

At that time, the management of traumatized patients was very disorganized, primitive and inefficient. Nobody wanted to stay in that kind of hospital if they could help it. I went there and found that they did not allow visits to any patients. Wearing my white lab coat, I decided to act very confident and just walk through the main door without asking questions—a strategy that usually worked in those years in Mexico. Sure enough, I entered the big room where many sick and injured people were on stretchers on the floor, screaming and scattered in various places—some of them bleeding, others being sutured. Somewhere in that huge room, I discovered my aunt. She was throwing up, resting on a stretcher, but she was coherent. When she saw me, she started crying very much, "Please, Alberto, take me away from here!"

The Red Cross doctors had already lavaged her stomach; they were just observing her to be sure that she fully recovered. I examined her and asked questions to be certain that she was fully awake and rational before I decided to take her home. In order to take a patient out of that hospital, the doctors had to discharge them under their responsibility or a fully trained, licensed doctor was required to sign a document, legally taking responsibility of the patient. The document had to be signed in front of the hospital's lawyers. I was not licensed, so that was out of the question. I decided to find the doctors that were in charge of my aunt and ask them to discharge her.

On the floor, I noticed a few young doctors. I interrupted their work and asked to speak with them. I introduced myself as a last year medical student from the Military Medical School and I perceived that they did not like my interruption. I explained the problem and requested them to examine my aunt to confirm that she was fully recovered so she could be officially discharged. They said that they would make rounds the next morning and wait until then to decide. If I wanted to take her home that night, they told me to go to the legal department and sign the required documents. I explained to them that I was not fully licensed because I was in the last year of medical school. They turned away, saying they could do nothing more for me.

I begged, "I am asking you for this favor because you are doctors. We're in the same profession. You can see my aunt, she is fully recovered. Please, discharge her. You are sending me to the legal office where there is nothing I can do."

All they could do was apologize.

Rather sad and feeling almost defeated, I had no choice but to go to a rather hostile territory: the legal office. I hoped I could do something. Sometimes in Mexico, things could be arranged in a rather roundabout way. In the office was a lady secretary behind a desk. In the back room the sound of glasses, ice and wagering could be discerned: a group was playing cards and having drinks.

"Can I speak to the lawyer in charge?"

The secretary replied, "What kind of business do you have?"

"It is a personal business."

She went inside the room, interrupted the card game and returned, asking me to wait a few minutes for the lawyer to come. About 30 minutes later, the lawyer came out. When I saw him, I saw a familiar face. It happened to be a lieutenant colonel lawyer, grandfather of Manuelito, my patient at the Central Military Hospital. This lawyer was moonlighting, working in the legal office of the Mexican Red Cross at night. He recognized me, "Dr. Peña, what are you doing here?" I explained the whole drama and he said, "There is no problem. Come with me."

We both walked back into the hospital, passing by the young doctors who refused to help me. They watched as the lawyer and I walked toward my aunt—their eyes and mouths open with incredulity. The lawyer called an ambulance and ordered them to transport my aunt to any place that I determined. The Mexican Red Cross was in charge of transporting patients from the place of accidents to their hospital, but never back. After being discharged, patients were required to ride in private ambulances to other hospitals or simply go by their own transportation. Yet, the lawyer ordered my aunt to be transported back to her home in a Red Cross ambulance. He was loud giving the orders.

Suddenly, one of the young doctors, very upset interrupted, "Excuse me, Sir. We have not discharged the patient. She cannot go home."

The lawyer spoke even louder, "I *said* this lady is going home in one of our ambulances with Dr. Peña and that is an order."

The young doctor felt more and more upset and impotent, "Sir, this person you call doctor is only a medical student. He is not fully licensed."

"Young man, I am in charge of the legal department. *This* is none of your business!"

I was there, in the middle of this discussion, making serious efforts not to smile. To the chagrin of the bureaucratically oriented doctors, my aunt was carried toward the ambulance, followed by the lawyer and I, chatting about Manuelito.

PEDRITO

In the summer of 1980, the Mexican army ordered me to travel to the northwest state of Sinaloa, more specifically, to the capital city of Culiacan. There, an army task force, called Condor, had been commissioned in the Sierra Madre Mountains to fight drug trafficking. Condor covered an enormous area with huge mountains, vast canyons, rivers and woods. At that time, the Sierra Madre was particularly convenient for international gangs to grow marijuana and opium. The gangs detected areas to grow the plants, near small rivers, hidden between the mountains. They built tiny improvised airstrips for their little planes and took seeds of the drug-producing plants and looked for local peasants to help them. A local peasant made around $2,000 per year growing corn but the drug lords offered 10 times more money just to care for their plants. After a certain number of months, the gangs returned in their little

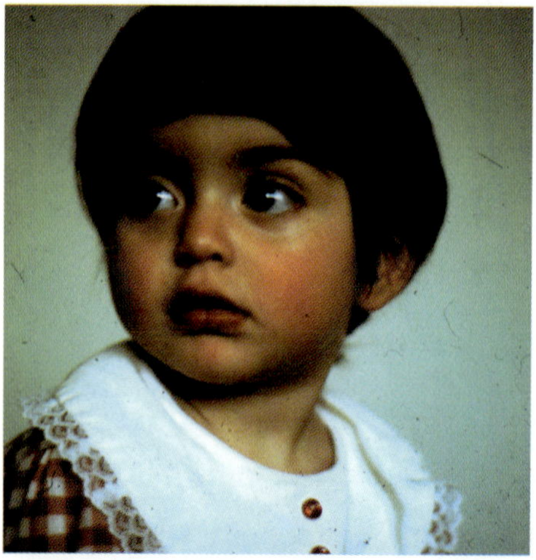

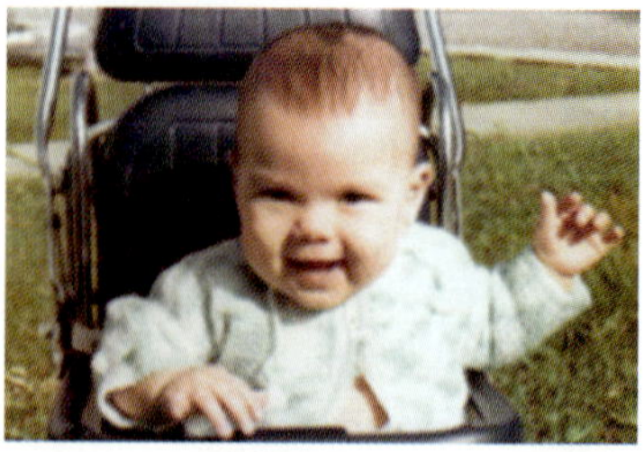

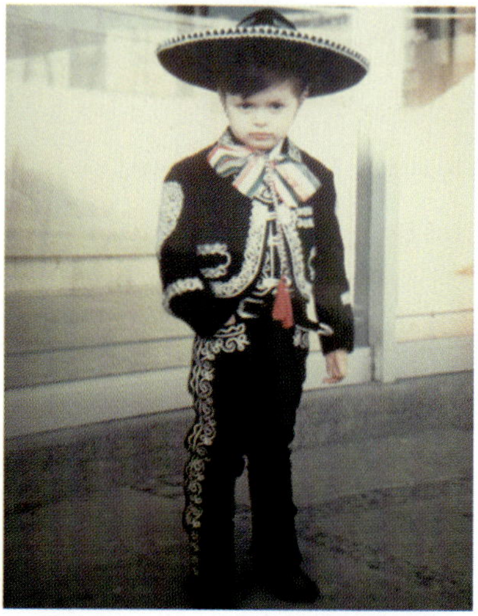

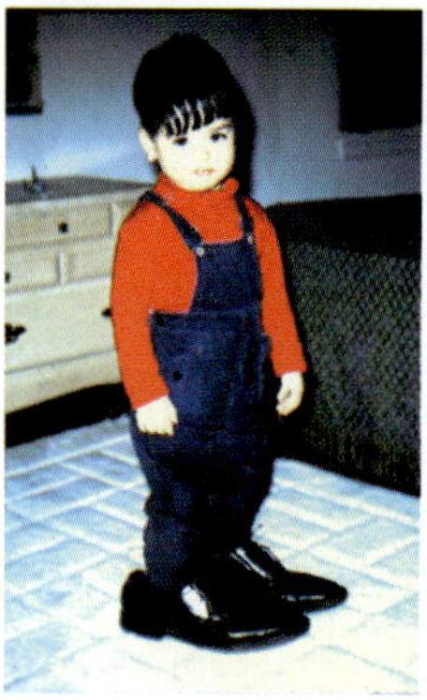

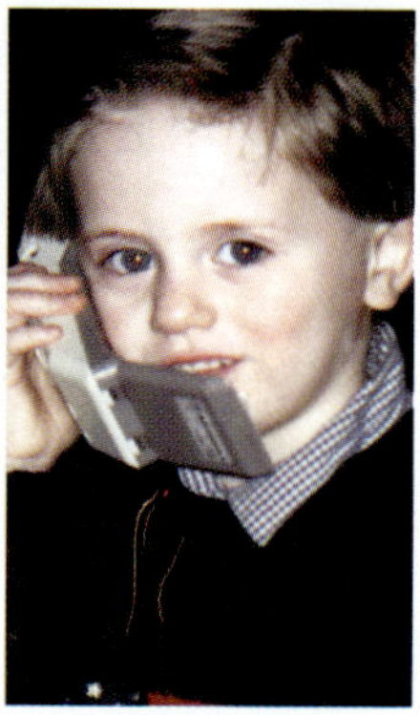

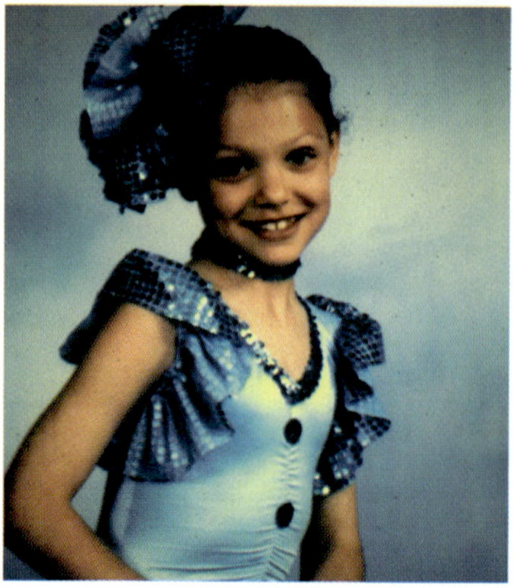

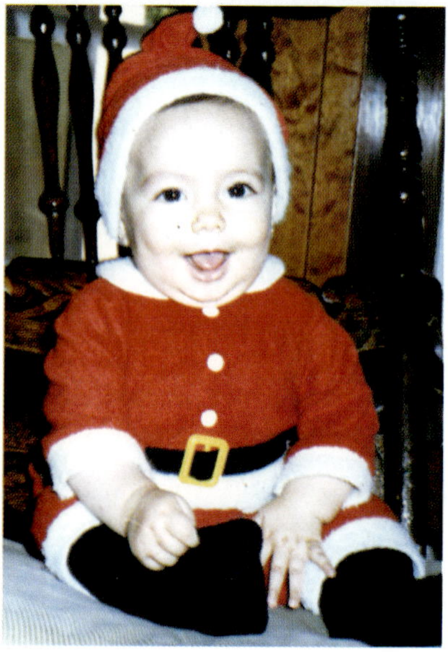

planes to take the drugs away. The drug traffickers' strategy was to stay on the move from one place to another. When the army searched in one area, the traffickers moved to another. If the army put too much pressure on them, they went to a completely different part of the country, making the army's mission nearly impossible.

The task force had to spread thousands of soldiers throughout the mountains, searching for marijuana and opium fields. In the process, they jailed the peasants who collaborated with the drug lords. Sometimes it happened peacefully, sometimes violently. The locals resented the army because, at times, they would kill one of their families. The Mexican army wanted to improve its image among the civilians in those conflicting areas. To do that, they sent doctors with specific instructions, to not only care for the soldiers (who almost never needed any care because they could be easily evacuated to big cities), but also the civilian population, providing medical care to every person requesting it. Doctors like me, were sent for a period of two or three weeks, leaving all of our affairs unattended, including private offices and academic obligations.

My ex-resident and now prominent pediatric surgeon, Dr. Victor Avila, was living in Culiacan at the time. He had been appointed chief of surgery of a small new children's hospital that was operated by the governor's wife. When I knew that I would be nearby, I called him and said that I would stop for a few hours. It would be nice to visit with him before going into the mountains. I was happy to see that he was working under good circumstances in a not very elegant, but very fine hospital.

The truth was that I was not very excited about spending two or three weeks in a rather isolated area, tending to civilian patients with skin rashes, bellyaches and colds. I knew I would miss operating on children and babies. I confided all of that in my conversation with Dr. Avila. He smiled and said he would do something about it.

From Culiacan, the army flew us by helicopter to a designated post in the middle of the Sierra Madre. Each doctor stayed with a group of about 30 soldiers and a couple of officers. Every morning, the soldiers went for long excursions, scouring the area for drug fields. Occasionally, they came back with a peasant responsible for cultivating the plants. The prisoner stayed in the improvised military barracks until a helicopter returned two or three weeks later. In the meantime, the prisoner was blindfolded because they did not want him to see the faces of the military personnel to avoid future retaliation. When the next helicopter arrived, the soldiers took the humble peasant to jail in Culiacan, only to see them liberated a few months later. The drug lords were never in the mountains, so the army could not arrest them. Everybody knew that the true responsibility for the drugs did not rest on the peasants but on the international drug rings and, most importantly, those who bought and used the drugs.

Interestingly, in 1677, a talented Mexican nun poet, Sor Juana Ines de la Cruz, wrote a poem in defense of women, more specifically in defense of prostitutes. What she said seems to be applicable to the modern problem of drugs:

Who is more sinful, the one who commits a sin to get the pay, or the one who pays to commit the sin?

Once I was in the mountains, surrounded by beautiful pine trees, I had time to read, to meditate and relax—things I could rarely do in the big city. The landscape was beautiful and it was an abrupt disconnection from my everyday, giving me a chance to think calmly and put things in perspective.

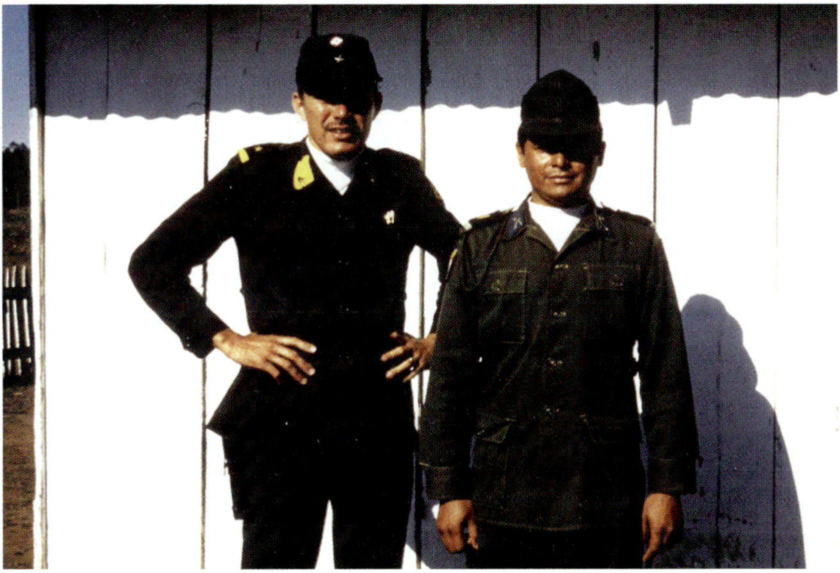

Dr. Peña in the mountains of Sierra Madre

A couple of days passed and the officer in charge asked if I would like to join them on a routine exploration. I enthusiastically accepted. He recommended that I bring a gun.

"Why should I bring a gun?"

The officer remarked, "You are a military person and nobody knows that you are a doctor. They may shoot at you and find out that you were a doctor after you died."

Three hours later, sure enough, in a little valley near a small river, a couple of individuals were spotted cultivating marijuana. The soldiers surrounded the area and started shooting. The two farmers ran in a panic and disappeared in a matter of seconds. Fortunately, nobody was wounded.

Walking back to camp that afternoon, the captain inquired, "What would you have done if we had injured one of those individuals?"

"I would do my best to save his life."

To which he smirked, "Don't worry, Dr. Peña. In this war there are no wounded prisoners."

After about 10 days in the mountains, a baby was born in Culiacan and was taken to the hospital where Victor Avila worked. The baby, Pedrito, had a serious defect of his abdominal wall called omphalocele,[111] which demanded an urgent, specialized operation. Consequently, Victor spoke to the governor's wife. He explained that I was the person who could benefit the baby the most and urged her to notify Condor's commander, requesting that I be brought to Culiacan to operate on Pedrito.

One morning I was sitting in the woods working on an

111 Congenital abdominal defect in which the intestine is outside of the abdomen.

improvised desk made out of old wood boxes, when I thought I heard the distant sound of a helicopter. I thought it was only my imagination since the army helicopter was not expected for a week later. However, the noise became more obvious and suddenly there was a federal police helicopter approaching our place. The pilots had a written order from the general commander of Condor to transport me back to Culiacan. Pedrito was waiting for me to operate on him. I could not believe that my friend Victor Avila had so much power, although it was actually Pedrito who had the true power. I jumped into the helicopter, went back to Culiacan and operated on the newborn baby. Victor Avila also organized a symposium of pediatric surgery for local pediatricians in addition to some social events.

LUPITA

Lupita was born with a form of esophageal defect that basically requires the total replacement of the esophagus with another portion of the gastrointestinal tract. In her case, I used a portion of her own colon. It was a long, technically demanding operation, but it was successful. For a period of time the new esophagus cannot be used; so, these patients are fed through a tube left in the stomach, coming out the abdominal wall. This is known as gastrostomy. Several weeks later a radiologic study is performed to confirm the integrity of the repair, determining if the patient can eat by mouth or needs a dilatation of any narrow portion of the replaced esophagus.

In Mexico, when a patient belonged to a poor family and it was thought that it would be a hardship for the family to care for them, it was frequently decided to keep the patient in the hospital until they had recovered enough to live in an environment with limited resources. That was the case of Lupita. However, her mother insisted that she could tend to the gastrostomy. I gave up and decided to trust the mother but not without some hesitation. So, I insisted that I wanted to see Lupita back in my clinic every week.

I was very disappointed when Lupita and her mother did not show up the following week. My colleagues and I were even more distraught when two months passed without any contact from Lupita and her family.

About three months after the operation, unexpectedly, Lupita and her family returned to the hospital. I was terribly upset and ready to reprehend Lupita's mother but the first thing that caught my eye was that Lupita actually looked healthy and happy. The mother apologized and explained everything. Shortly after Lupita was discharged from the hospital, she was abducted and disappeared. The police were notified and they had been looking for the criminals for months. Finally, the police apprehended them and put them in jail, reuniting the family. Our social services department confirmed her story. Amazingly, the couple that abducted Lupita took exceptional care of her. The gastrostomy tube was intact. Lupita was eating everything by mouth and was gaining weight.

GIANNINA

I had the privilege of operating on this little girl at Ospedale Pediatrico Bambino Gesù, a children's hospital located in Vatican City. Giannina's operation went well. During the procedure there was a conversation about the Sistine Chapel. With a hidden intention, I shared with my host pediatric surgeons that I only had a previous opportunity to visit that magnificent place and contemplate Michelangelo's masterful work but that was many years before and, unfortunately, it was too crowded then. I told them that I heard that the Sistine Chapel had been recently restored. "It must be beautiful," I pondered. "I would love to see it again."

My Italian colleagues talked between themselves but I could not understand what they were saying. About 30 minutes later, one of them walked into the operation room, "Dr. Peña, this afternoon the Sistine Chapel is closed. However, as a special consideration for you, at 3:00 p.m., a guide will take you inside!"

I finished the operation of Giannina and hurried to the Sistine Chapel, escorted by one of my generous hosts. Coincidentally, watching my operation was a good friend of mine, a German pediatric surgeon and prominent embryologist, Dr. Dietrich Kluth. I asked him to stay close to me and he participated and enjoyed this magnificent affair. Dietrich, the guide and I spent almost two hours alone inside the Sistine Chapel. We spread out on the floor to admire the frescoes of the ceiling. What a breath-holding inspirational experience!

At the end of our private tour, I was notified that a couple of Swiss Guards would lead us through the building to the Saint Peter Cathedral. As I was enjoying the whole event, I felt a great deal of gratitude toward Giannina, the little patient who allowed all of this to happen. I had the opportunity to rejoice! Bringing back my experience in my mind when I visited my very Catholic mother, I detailed the whole event and gave her a silver rosary from the Vatican.

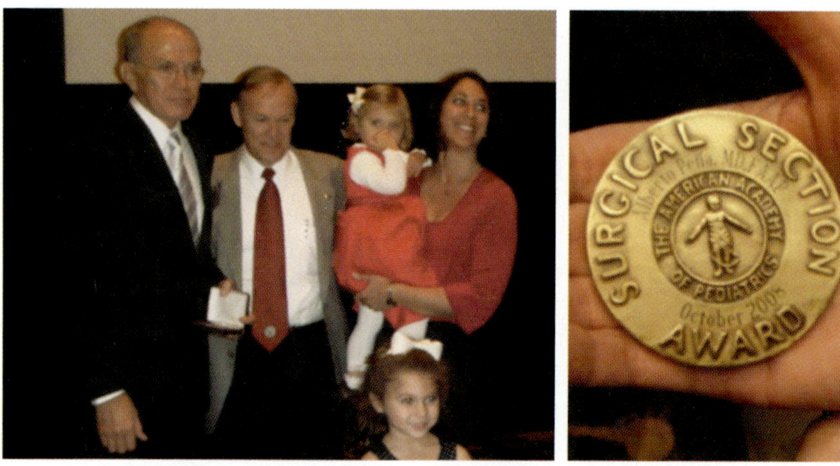

Left: With Dr. Richard Ricketts, President, Surgical Section, American Academy of Pediatrics, with beautiful Nina and her lovely mother and sister; William Ladd medal ceremony, Boston 2008; Right: The William Ladd Medal

NINA

Nina is a beautiful girl. I had the pleasure of operating on her and watching her grow happy and nurtured by a loving family.

The Surgical Section of the American Academy of Pediatrics presented me the most important distinction given every year to honor a pediatric surgeon for their contributions to pediatric surgery: the William Ladd Medal. I felt extremely honored and privileged. It was one of the happiest days of my life. I felt gratitude towards my American colleagues and a sense of responsibility to improve my performance as a surgeon. During the ceremony, I was happily surprised when little Nina walked into the big conference room and presented me with the famous medal. Thank you, Nina!

JULIETTE

When I was a child in elementary school, I was introduced to a very special museum. It is a castle located on top of a hill in the middle of Mexico City. It is called Castillo de Chapultepec (Chapultepec Castle). It is a place that plays a very important role in Mexico's history. Through many years, the castle served several purposes, including being the Mexican military academy during the American invasion in 1847. In fact, it was the last point of resistance of the Mexican army during the war. Six young cadets died in the defense of the bastion. They are very revered national heroes in Mexico. Later on, the castle became the official presidential residence.

In 1860, the president of Mexico was Benito Juarez; born in the state of Oaxaca, he was the first pure Zapoteco Indian to become president of Mexico. At that time, there was a great deal of racial discrimination in Mexico. Nobody expected that a very humble Indian would rise to become the president of the country. He is, up to now, perhaps the most revered figure in Mexican history.

In those years, the Catholic Church played an important role in the Mexican government. They owned an enormous amount of land and fortune—nothing could be done without the Church's approval. Benito Juarez decided, for the first time, to separate the government from the church and confiscated all of the Church's properties. This prompted a bloody civil war known as Guerra de Reforma (Reform War). All of the conservatives and Church leaders joined against Benito Juarez. The very conservative, rich Catholics believed it would be better for Mexico to be governed by a European prince. They thought that Mexico was not ready to be a democratic republic. Mexico was a very young country and was very difficult to govern. There was a significant amount of corruption and many coups, presidents changed very often and a few decades before, as a consequence of a war, Mexico lost half of its territory to the United States.

Due to all of these circumstances, plus the economical problems, Benito Juarez declared a moratorium in the payment of the foreign debt. The most affected countries were Spain, England and France and so they decided to invade Mexico. However, England and Spain backed out in the last minutes. Napoleon III, at that time the King of France, had his own agenda and sent his army to invade Mexico. In the first attempt, the Mexican army defeated the French army at Puebla on May 5, 1862. (Mexican's celebrate this as Cinco de Mayo.) However, the French army went back to Veracruz, received significant amount of reinforcements and eventually invaded Mexico. Benito Juarez had to flee Mexico City with part of the national treasure and ministers. They traveled all over the country organizing guerrilla warfare against the French.

The Catholic Church and the conservative Mexicans were very pleased by the invasion and saw the chance to bring a European prince to install a monarchy in Mexico. Napoleon III offered the throne of Mexico to Maximilian, the brother of Francis Joseph, emperor of the Austrian-Hungarian Empire. Maximilian was a young prince and was married to Charlotte, the daughter of King Leopold I of Belgium. The young couple lived in Miramar, at the border of Italy with what later became Yugoslavia. They had a small beautiful castle in front of the Adriatic Sea.

Maximilian and Charlotte received the invitation and hesitated for some time. Maximilian requested several thousands of signatures of prominent Mexicans to demonstrate that the people really wanted him. The Mexican conservatives did not hesitate to obtain thousands of signatures. A very prominent group of conservatives even traveled to Miramar to offer Maximilian the "throne of Mexico." Maximilian and Charlotte accepted and made all of the necessary preparations to go to Mexico with the support of Napoleon III, who offered to maintain his army in Mexico for a few years until Maximilian raised his own army and pacified the country. The emperor of Austria, Francis Joseph, also promised to help his brother, provided he resigned his right to the throne of Austria—if Francis Joseph died, Maximilian was next in line to the throne. Possibly out of greed or even fear, Maximilian's own brother asked him to resign that privilege.

After several months of preparations, the young couple finally took the long trek from Miramar to Veracruz, Mexico and from there to Chapultepec Castle in Mexico City. Prior to their arrival, everything was prepared for them in the castle, including the décor, simulating the Austrian style with all of its pomp and elegance. When they arrived at the castle, they were welcomed by all of the conservatives.

Meanwhile, Benito Juarez was still running a guerrilla war against the French and the country was not completely pacified. Juarez was mainly operating in the north of the country, occasionally crossing the border into the United States. On a specific occasion, he had to move to New Orleans to work in a cigar factory and from there he sailed down to Acapulco to continue fighting.

Maximilian sent a letter to Benito Juarez offering him to become one of his ministers. Benito Juarez, very dignified, answered the letter by apologizing for his delayed response because he was "very busy with his job as president of Mexico." As the legally elected president, he was not in a position to accept Maximilian's proposal and he proclaimed that he would let history judge and pronounce the final verdict of all of these unfair series of events.

Maximilian, who happened to be more liberal than expected, did not fulfill the expectations of the conservatives and the Catholic

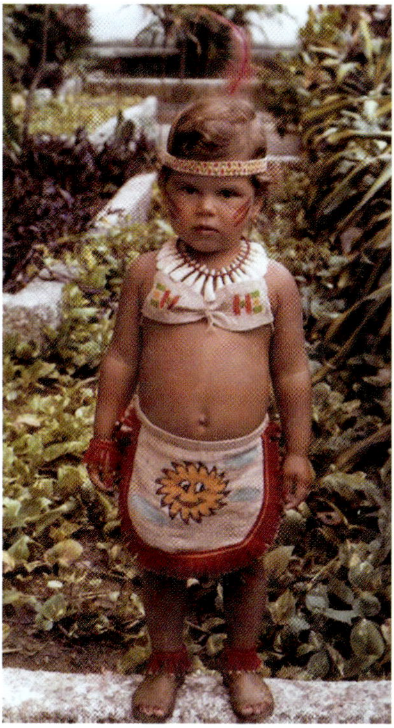

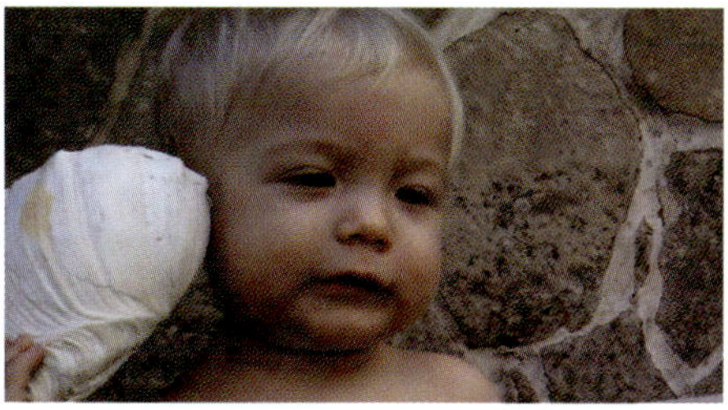

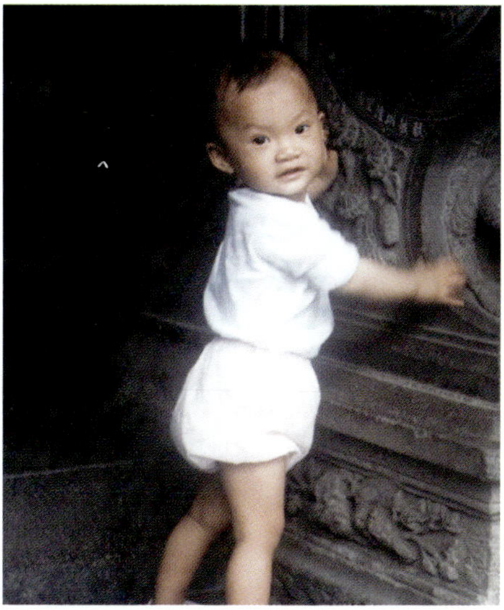

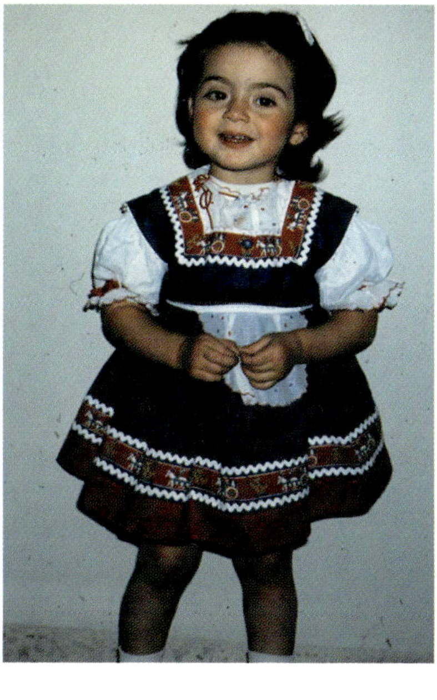

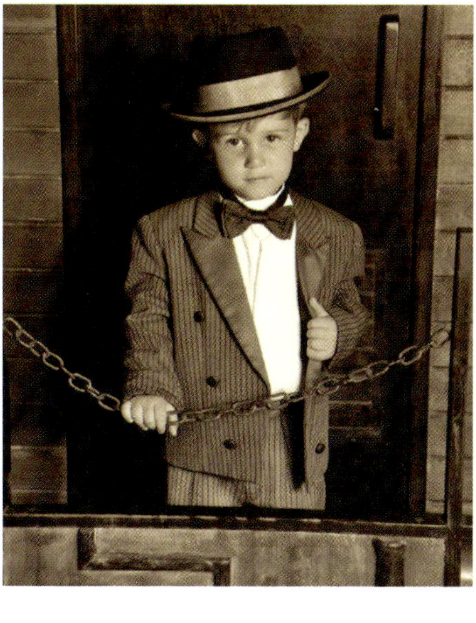

Church in Mexico. After a short period of time, about 2 or 3 years, Napoleon III had to pull the majority his army out of Mexico because he was fighting his own wars in Europe. In addition, Maximilian's brother refused to send additional troops to Mexico. The guerilla army of Benito Juarez started growing. Maximilian was offered exile but he decided to remain as "emperor of Mexico" and defend his throne to the end. This is a sad story because Maximilian actually turned out to be more idealistic than expected and he took his role as emperor and "savior of Mexico" very seriously, whereas, for the majority of Mexicans, he was another invader. Juarez's army continued to advance, surrounding the center of Mexico. Maximilian moved to a city called Queretaro and commanded his army with three loyal Mexican generals: Miramon, Mejia and Marquez. Again, he was repeatedly offered to leave the country but he refused.

Commanded by Benito Juarez and General Mariano Escobedo, the guerilla army continued, finally defeating the imperial army. They took Maximilian and his loyal Mexican generals as prisoners. They were judged and sentenced to death. Many European governments protested and begged Benito Juarez to pardon Maximilian but he decided to proceed and the four individuals were executed in Cerro de las Campanas, Queretaro, Mexico.

During the guerilla war, Charlotte fled Mexico looking for help in Europe. She first went to France where Napoleon III did not welcome her. She pleaded with her cousin, Napoleon's wife, begging for help but they did not support her. From there, she went to Rome to talk to the pope, seeking refuge. She stayed one night, because while she was talking to the pope, she started showing symptoms of mental deterioration. It is said that she is the only woman who has ever slept in the Vatican. She never recovered and became a psychiatric patient, went back to Belgium and died in 1929, full of fantasies and dreams. The body of Maximilian was embalmed, sent back to Europe and buried in one of the cathedrals in Vienna.

When I was a child, I visited the Chapultepec Castle and saw that it was still decorated in the way Maximilian and Charlotte intended. There were very delicate china, porcelain objects, chandeliers, furniture, fancy tapestry, elegant uniforms and swords, all made in the European style. Huge paintings of the very attractive young Emperor next to his beautiful princess were mounted on the walls. Maximilian's luxury carriage, covered with gold on the outside and silk inside, was also on display. The Mexican government decided to put Benito Juarez's official carriage next to Maximilian's luxury carriage to show the contrast between the extravagance and richness of Maximilian with the draconian, humble vehicle used by the Mexican president.

*****

Many years later, I was invited to northern Italy to operate on several children. I realized that I was very near Miramar, the place where Maximilian and Charlotte lived before going to Mexico and I asked my hosts, if it would be possible for me to visit. I was taken and was very impressed by the beauty of the little castle situated on a cliff overlooking the Adriatic. While Maximilian and Charlotte were preparing the trip to Mexico, they had Mexican paintings and decorative motifs displayed throughout the castle. There was a big painting depicting the moment in which they boarded a frigate called La Novara, which took them to Mexico directly from Miramar. I enjoyed that trip very much.

More years passed. When I was living in New York, I received a letter from the Belgium Consulate. The consul of Belgium in New York, on behalf of Princess Lillian, invited me to Belgium to operate on a little girl by the name of Juliette who was born with a complex cloaca. Princess Lillian was the widow of King Leopold III of Belgium. Leopold III was the son of Leopold II. Leopold II was the brother of Charlotte. Both, Charlotte and Leopold II were children of Leopold I. Little Juliette was the daughter of one of the security guards of Princess Lillian. The security guard told the princess about this unfortunate event and she decided to investigate what a cloaca was.

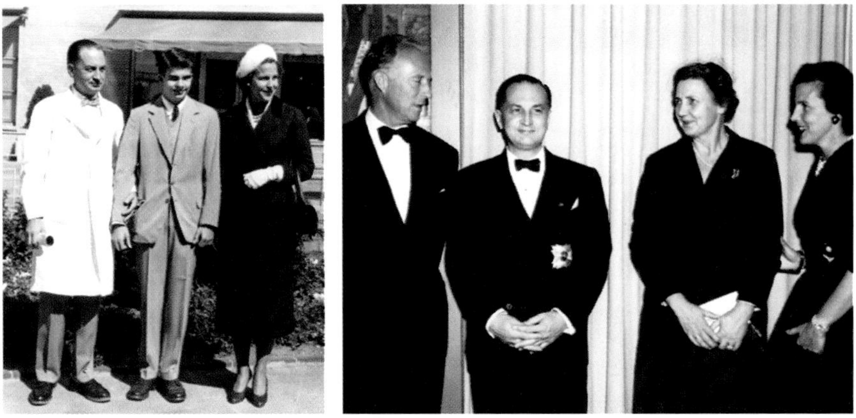

Left: Dr. Robert Gross with his patient and Princess Lillian; Right: Leopold III, King of Belgium, Dr. Robert Gross (decorated), Mrs. Gross, and Princess Lillian

The first thing she did was to call her friend, Dr. Michael de Bakey in Texas. Michael de Bakey and Princess Lillian had met many years before because her child was born with a cardiovascular malformation called aortic coarctation. When the child was an adolescent, Princess Lillian and Leopold III went to Boston to have Dr. Robert Gross, creator of the technique to operate aortic coarctations, operate on their son. Dr. Gross operated on the child successfully. Subsequently, Leopold the III invited Dr. Gross to Belgium and decorated him. After that experience, Princess Lillian decided to create a foundation to help children born with cardiac malformations. As an advisor, she selected Dr. Michael de Bakey, a prominent cardiac surgeon from Texas. They became good friends and they brought many children with cardiac conditions from poor countries to be operated on in the United States.

Princess Lillian was shocked when she heard that Dr. de Bakey did not know about a cloaca. Then she went to the dictionary and found that a cloaca is the sewage of ancient cities. Another entry defined cloaca as the single orifice that birds have to pass waste and for reproductive purposes. Finally, after much investigation, Belgian doctors explained to the princess that it is also the name given to a malformation that occurs in girls and they told her that I was the person to call. I accepted the invitation and we set up a date. I communicated with the Belgian doctors concerning the technical aspects of the trip. My Belgian colleagues took advantage of my trip (paid for by the princess) and brought more patients with similar conditions to see if I could also repair them. Of course, I accepted.

I traveled to Belgium. At the airport, there was a car waiting for me with a chauffeur. I thought he would take me to a hotel. To my surprise, he took me to the palace at Argenteuil, outside Brussels, which was the official residence of Princess Lillian. I arrived at the estate and they took me to my quarters. It was morning but I had to rest because I traveled overnight. They told me that Princess Lillian would wait for me for lunch.

Later that day, I went to the dining room and there was Princess Lillian seated at one extreme of the table, about 20 feet away from me. Next to the princess was a huge dog that barked dangerously and threateningly every time I moved. She and I had a very pleasant lunch.

At that time, Princess Lillian was in her 70s and was still a very attractive woman. We had conversations on many subjects and I realized that I was talking to someone with a vast education and culture. She was fluent in several languages. She told me about her son born with an aortic coarctation and how she and the king met Dr. Gross. Then, I explained that I trained with Dr. Gross, I admired him and he was one of my mentors. We talked about many subjects related to Boston. She offered me some photographs and letters related to her trip to Boston, which I gladly accepted. After our first acquaintance, I was taken to the hospital to see the babies that I would operate on, including Juliette.

In the following three days, the routine was to have breakfast and a nice conversation with Princess Lillian and then her car would take me to the hospital. I was back late in the afternoon, took a short rest and then had dinner with Princess Lillian. On the third day, she invited very prominent Belgian doctors for dinner. I felt more confident with the Princess by then and told her that as a child I used to visit the Chapultepec Castle because I was very impressed by the story of Maximilian and Charlotte.

"Are you really interested in that? In our family, Charlotte was very important and we frequently talk about her. She was my husband's aunt and he liked her very much. She lived in another castle nearby and my husband used to visit her during the weekends. Sometimes he found her perfectly normal and rational, showing signs of her high intellect. Other times, he found her

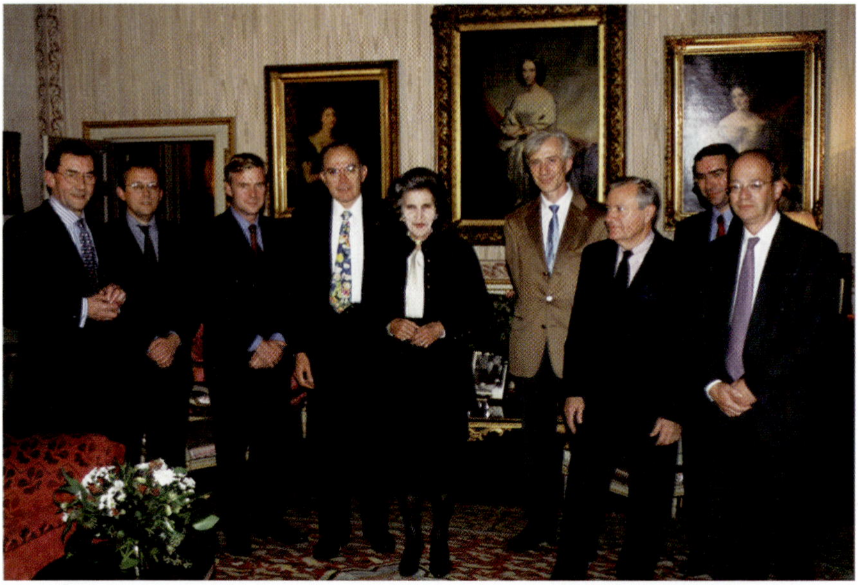

Dinner at the Palace of Argenteuil, Brussels with Princess Lillian and prominent Belgium surgeons: Professors Otte, Reding, Rubay, Alberto Peña, Princess Lillian, Verellen, Sluisman, Vliers, and Wese

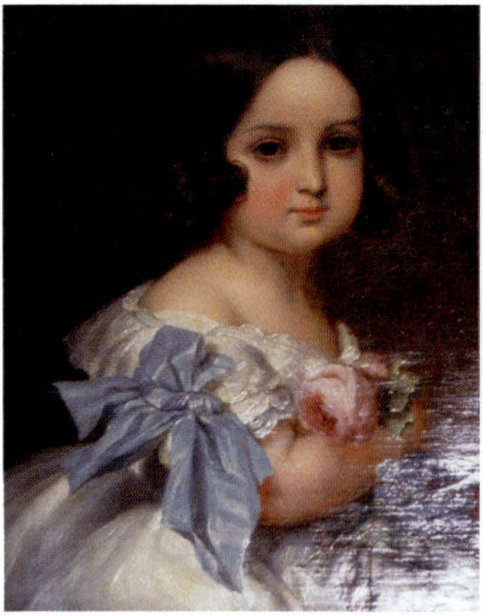

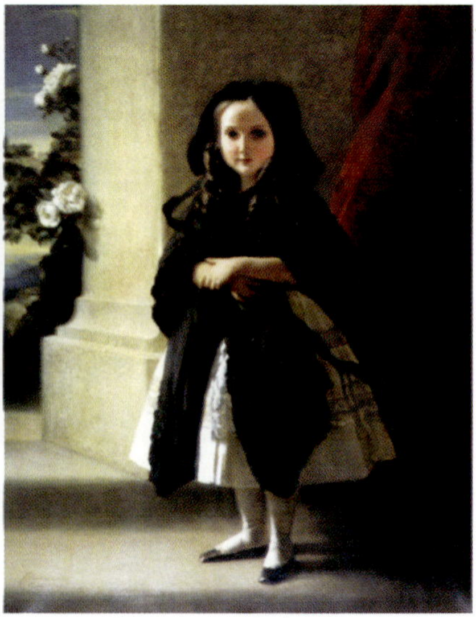

Left: Charlotte at age 2; Right: Charlotte at age 5

spraying water on the carpet, saying that she was watering the flowers. If you are interested in Charlotte, I will be able to show you many more things about her tomorrow when you return. I will ask my secretary to get ready. Don't forget your camera."

The next day after dinner, we walked through the castle and she showed me paintings of Charlotte as a baby, when she was 3 years old and when she was 6 years old. She was actually a beautiful girl. Finally, she took me to a special room where she had many valuable things. "I am going to give you something very special, Dr. Peña." She opened a box and showed me a bracelet. The bracelet belonged to Maria Louise, Charlotte's mother. Maria Louise gave the bracelet to Charlotte and she wore it all her life. Princess Lillian said that when Charlotte died, the family debated whether they should keep the bracelet on her wrist or take it away from her. They decided to take it. I looked at the bracelet—it was beautiful. To my surprise, Princess Lillian held out the bracelet, "Please, take it home with you."

The next day Princess Lillian surprised me again with a bunch of letters that belonged to the Charlotte's private file. The letters were written when she was still in Mexico and was asking for money from Belgium, because the economic situation of Mexico was not very good. Basically, the Mexican empire was falling apart. Princess Lillian also gave me several photographs of Dr. Gross, the King of Belgium, herself, and her 15-year-old son in the little garden in the center of Children's Hospital Boston.

I treasure these things.

When it was time to say goodbye, I thanked little Juliette for her great power, the magnificent experience and wonderful privileges that were granted to me. I went back to Mexico with Charlotte's bracelet, many of her letters and photographs of Dr. Gross and the king of Belgium. I like to think that this is a small world: Because a little girl was born with a congenital malformation, life brought together a Mexican child dreaming at the Chapultepec Castle, a princess and relative of Charlotte, Dr. Gross and the king of Belgium.

TOÑO

Toño was born in to a privileged family in Mexico City. Antonio Lopez-Silames, his father, was a young, charismatic businessman and member of a prominent family that owned an important pharmaceutical company in Mexico. Maria Eugenia, Toño's mother, was a young, pretty lady, also very intelligent and a member of a prominent family as well. The child seemed to be healthy but within a few hours after birth, it became evident that something was wrong with him. He could not swallow saliva. Unfortunately, he was born with a malformation known as esophageal atresia. This defect consists in a congenital lack of continuity in the esophagus. The separation of the ends of the esophagus can be short and relatively easy to repair or very long, which even today, represents a serious surgical challenge.

In those years, the surgical treatment of that condition in Mexico was performed in two stages. During the newborn period, the blind esophagus was connected to the skin of the neck, which allowed the baby to swallow saliva and avoid aspiration into his lungs. In order for the baby to receive nutrition, it was necessary to create an opening in the abdominal wall communicating with the stomach. The baby received milk and food through this device, called gastrostomy tube. Babies grew up and usually two or three years later, when they were considered strong enough to tolerate a major procedure, they underwent an operation to replace the missing esophagus with a piece of their own intestine.

Toño's parents were fascinated with their first baby and took excellent care of him. Toño grew up as a charismatic, happy child surrounded by love. However, the parents knew that sooner or later, they would have to do something because he was becoming aware of his own abnormality. Finally, when Toño was approximately four years old, the parents accepted the proposal of a major repair to be done in Mexico City by the most important pediatric surgeon. The operation went on for many hours. The child survived the operation but had fever and obvious manifestations of infection in the following days. The operation failed. The piece of bowel that was interposed between the ends of the esophagus did not survive. After several days of suffering, struggling and major efforts from the doctors to improve his condition, Toño died. The young parents became adults and mature human beings within a few months of intense suffering. It was hard for them to understand why and how something like that could happen.

Time went by. They had other healthy children. But deep in inside remained the memory of their first child and the misery he endured. Several years after Toño died, Maria Eugenia and Antonio decided that possibly the most painful episode of their lives had a meaning and the short existence of Toño should transcend in some way. In a conversation with their pediatrician, they expressed a desire to do something meaningful to help children born with congenital malformations and their tormented parents.

The pediatrician knew me because I had the honor and privilege of operating on his patients. He suggested that the parents contact me. Antonio, the young father, and I met and had a long talk in very friendly terms. What we both had in common was the fact that our first sons were born with congenital malformations and both of them died at about the same age. Besides my personal experience as a pediatric surgeon, dealing with children born with congenital malformations, I could contribute my ideas for other ways to assist children and parents. Antonio, with his entrepreneurial mentality and organizational skills, plus his economical resources, could implement many of my thoughts and dreams. One of the first things Antonio decided to do was to organize a formal meeting of several prominent Mexican doctors, including geneticists and doctors dedicated to prenatal studies, as well as obstetricians.[112]

112 Physicians specializing in pregnancy, the care of the expectant woman and childbirth.

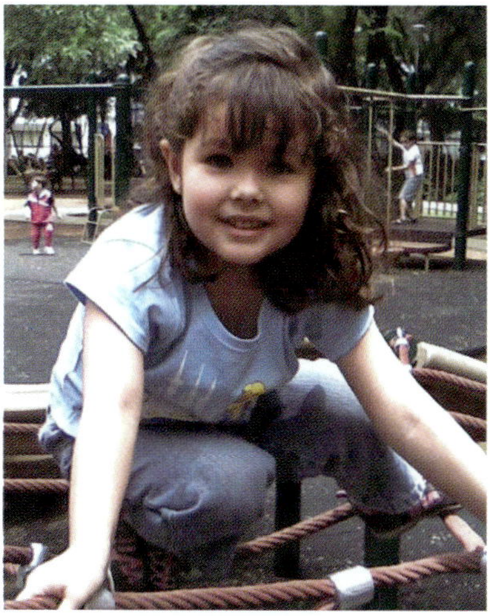

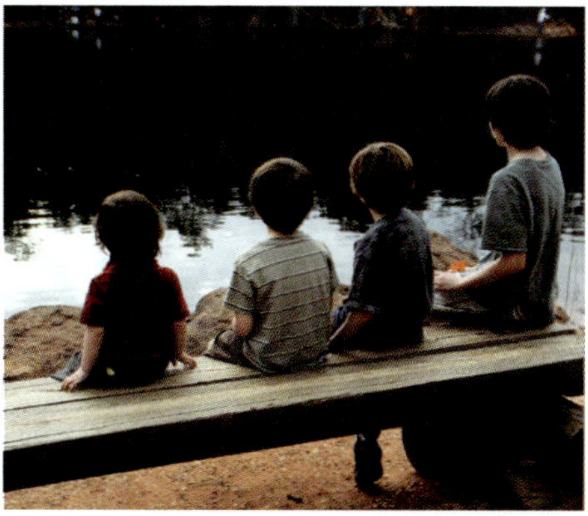

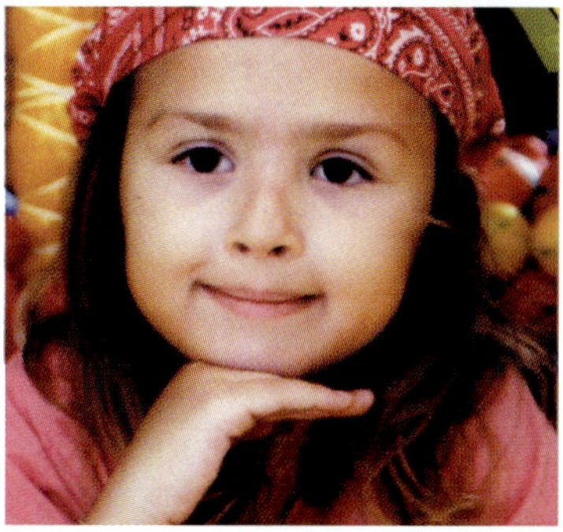

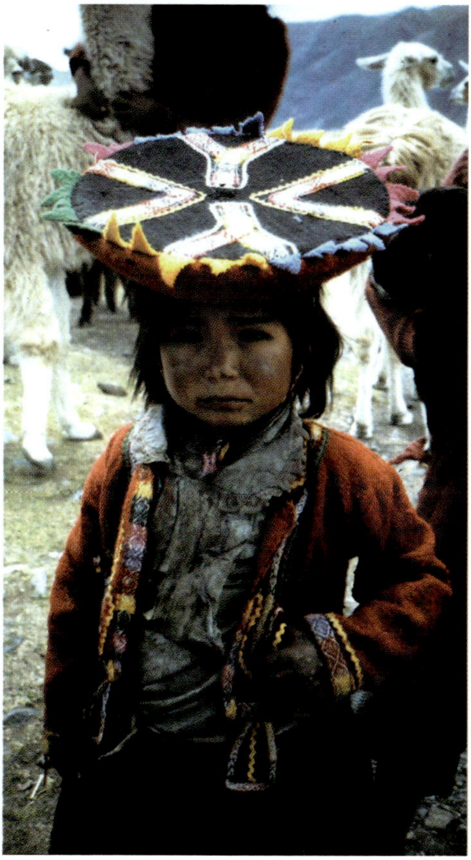

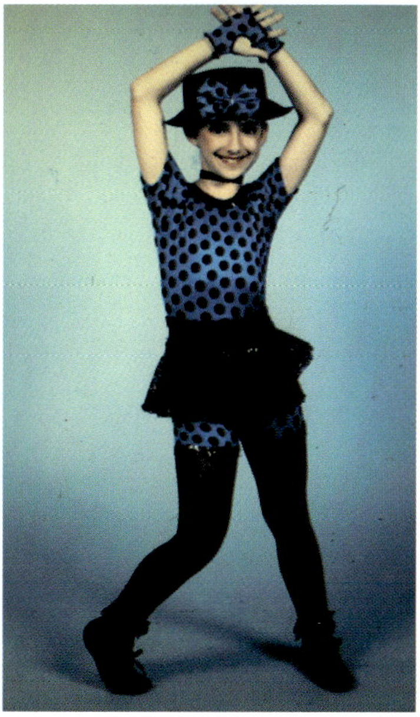

With the leadership of the American organization known as March of Dimes, this meeting was organized in Mexico City.

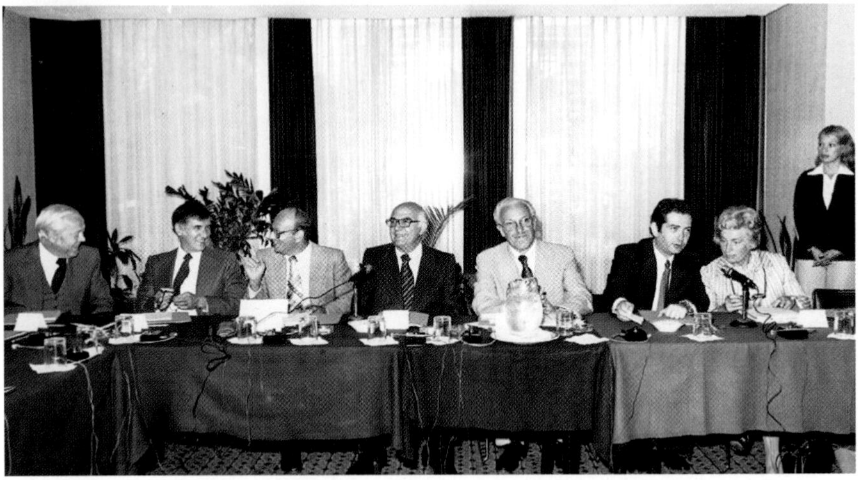

Antonio Lopez-Silanes, seated sixth from left, "March of Dimes" and Mexican health authorities; Creation of GEN Mexico

From the leaders of March of Dimes, we all learned many things and started forming this ambitious project. We were very astonished to find that the overwhelming majority of medical schools in Mexico had no formal teaching of genetics. Another very important action that Antonio decided to take was to establish a direct communication with Mexican public health authorities. Of course, they welcomed Antonio's initiative to promote the importance of prenatal care and the knowledge of genetics amongst doctors to increase the index of suspicion for the diagnoses and early treatment of congenital malformations. Antonio was particularly interested in the prevention of congenital malformations. The statistics showed that an enormous majority of Mexican mothers did not receive any prenatal care. I was the first doctor to work with Antonio and very soon we recruited a large number of prominent Mexican doctors of various disciplines, all related with congenital malformations, to aid in the project.

The organization was named GEN because of its obvious meaning (in Spanish, *gen* means gene). The letter "G" stands for *grupo* (group), "E" for *estudios* (studies) and "N" for *nacimiento* (which means birth). GEN became popular all over the country. In a short period of time, the organization paid our expenses to go and give lectures about genetics, prenatal diagnosis and early care of congenital malformations to every medical school in the country. The talks were given to medical students, to doctors of the community and to parents. The impact was enormous.

During those years, I dedicated myself to the study and treatment of anorectal malformations with a new approach. Antonio was particularly enthusiastic about my work. Because I was working in an anatomic area that was not particularly known within the community of surgeons, it was necessary to have the best possible audiovisual material. (This was in a time before videos.) Antonio was generous enough to pay for the making of a professional film, which I was able to present first at the American Pediatric Surgical Association Meeting in Phoenix, Arizona and, subsequently, all over the world.

I like to think that Little Antonio, as well as my son, Gustavo, had a very significant impact in the improvement of the quality of life for affected children and their parents, in Mexico and all over the world.

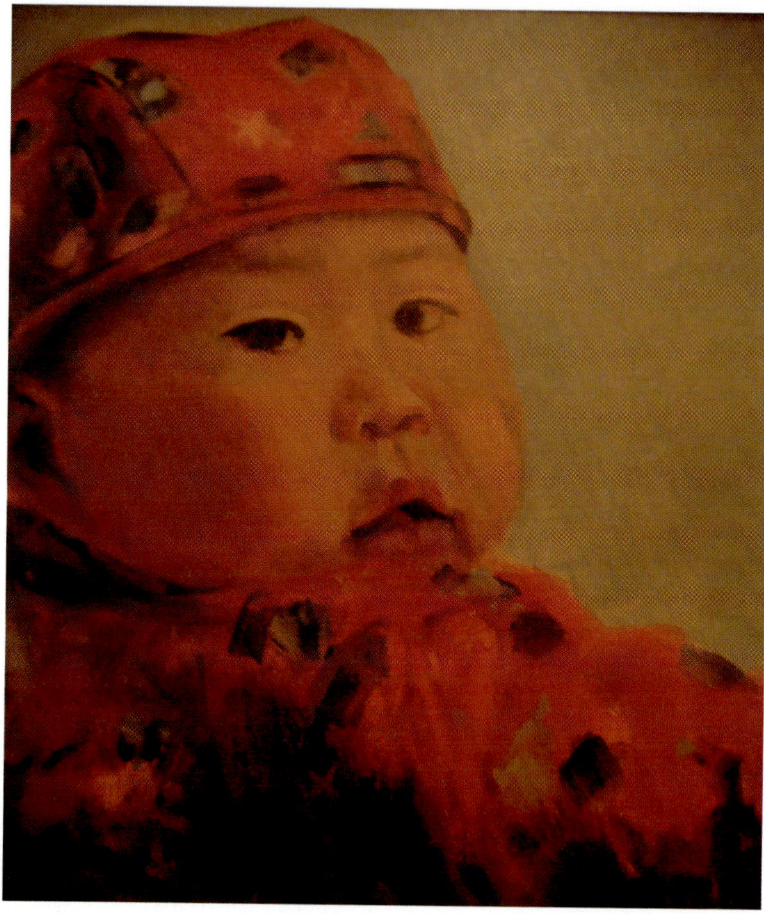

PUTTING THINGS INTO PERSPECTIVE: THE IMPORTANCE OF TRAVELING

As a consequence of the multiple pressures of an individual's environment, a general tendency of human beings is to center their attention and become overwhelmed and obsessed about everyday obstacles. Little by little, without even noticing, people develop the sense that the end of the world is the line of their horizon. They risk losing perspective and becoming increasingly incapable of putting things into a realistic context, forgetting that everything is relative. Half full or half empty: one can decide to look at individual predicaments in a pessimistic way or, rather, measure all the positive aspects of their life. Traveling can be a catalyst for such introspection.

Traveling abroad presents the possibility to meet people who speak different languages, practice different religions and have different habits and cultural histories—even their quality of life and existential concepts may be completely different. Feeling a bit overwhelmed, the traveler might long for the comfortable, planned, predictable, safe environment of his home. Alternatively, though, this is an occasion for him to learn more about where he is, the people's everyday problems, the various reactions that people with different values have and the idea of what happiness is to them. By doing so, a new dimension may be discovered and the traveler can now see himself from the outside.

Certainly, when contemplating the practice of medicine and surgery in the United States (from the outside), it is discovered just how privileged the country really is. A general characteristic of humans is also rediscovered: if not careful, people feel unhappy because of frivolous problems and they have a tendency to become upset about things that seem very serious, simply because there are no parameters of comparison.

It is always flattering for me to be invited to other countries to give lectures and operate on children. Throughout my travels I was fortunate to meet extraordinary people. I sometimes found myself operating under very rudimentary conditions in a very poor country and a few days later, I was operating in a fully equipped, sophisticated operating room, in an advanced country in some other part of the world. I knew that Mexico was a poor nation but I learned that "poor" was a relative concept because I visited countries that were much poorer.

There are many things to be gained from these "poor" societies.

People with limited and scant natural resources sometimes achieve a great deal of economical and technological development due to their discipline and work ethic. With this knowledge, one can develop more of a universal mind-set, becoming less nationalistic. In traveling, one finds common denominators among the diversity of human beings. I am extremely grateful to all those surgeons who were generous and brave enough to invite me to operate in their hospitals.

Travel is fatal to prejudice, bigotry, and narrow mindedness.
—Mark Twain

POLISH PARENTS

When I first visited Poland, during the time of the communist regime, I had the pleasure of operating at a children's hospital in Krakow, Poland. The doctors were extremely courteous, the nurses were dedicated and hard working and the children were beautiful. I operated on three children and from day one (following my usual routine), I expressed my desire to speak with their parents. I also requested the presence of a Polish surgical resident as a translator to describe what I did to their children, the type of care needed after the operation, the importance of long-term assessments and future consequences of the operation.

My hosts, Polish pediatric surgeons, were a little nervous and explained that it was extremely complicated to please me because the parents worked in a factory and they were not permitted to visit their children during weekdays. I was not intimidated and decided to challenge the system to the limit of my capacity. I acted this way out of curiosity and as a manifestation of my disagreement of not allowing the parents to visit their children. I pointed out that part of my teaching was to show the residents how to communicate with parents and how to discuss future evaluations of the patients. I expected the bureaucratic authorities to understand this; after all, it was for the benefit of the people.

During the following two days, I insisted upon my request and my hosts were growing more nervous, talking amongst themselves. I could not understand one word but I perceived the anxiety that I produced with my petition and their inability to please me. Finally, when I was just about to finish my third day operation, a smiling Polish doctor notified me that they were very happy because the authorities granted permission to bring the parents into the hospital! I was very pleased.

The parents were in the general director's office. I went downstairs with a surgical resident and found the three couples in a very large office, sitting on a sofa. Wearing the typical attire of factory workers, three rather nervous, humble couples were waiting for me. I sat in front of them with the translating resident. Couple by couple, I explained the malformations, the details of my operations and the care their children would require in the following days, weeks, months and years. In the middle of my description, the parents started crying. I stopped and asked the resident to inquire if had I said something wrong and why they were so upset. He replied that the parents were very moved to be called to the hospital during working hours to receive such a thorough explanation—something that they had never done before. While translating this to me, the resident was also crying.

Happiness is a state of mind.

INDIAN MOTHER

I have been to India several times. During one of the trips, I operated on a little boy with an anorectal malformation. As usual, when I finished, I requested to have a conversation with the child's parents using the help of a resident as translator. My request was granted and very soon I was sitting in front of the patient's mother. She was a very unassuming lady who did not look into my eyes. She was dressed in traditional Indian clothes and had beautiful facial features. I began by asking if she had other children. She said that she had three: the one I had just operated on, another afflicted with polio and a third in the hospital because she was extremely sick with severe burns on 60% of her body. Trying not to show my emotions, I described what I did to her son and the kind of attention that was needed. I gave her my card so we could correspond and explained that I would try to help her from abroad.

When I finished, I asked if she had any questions. She thought for a couple of minutes. She said that she already had a lot of trouble with the other two sick children, so as a gift, I should accept the child that I operated on. I should take him to my country and care for him. She would give him up because she knew that the child would be better off with me!

Prior to this, I had been exposed to poverty but never to the point in which a mother would give up a child for his benefit. After this kind of experience, it is extremely difficult for a surgeon to return to the United States and complain about the everyday "problems" of medicine and surgery. Fortunately, I grew up in a developing country and this helped me to maintain a certain degree of perspective about the so-called "problems" in America.

VISITING PROFESSORS

IMAN was not representative of the quality of medicine and surgery in the rest of Mexico. We had more resources than other little government hospitals; nevertheless, there were still many restrictions in terms of materials and equipment. Like in many other developing countries, we learned that medical equipment and materials considered disposable in developed countries, were 100 percent reusable in poor countries. It was that, or nothing. In the US, like in many other developed countries, electric cauteries[113] had disposable pads and cables with disposable pencils and needle tips. In Mexico, we used, used and reused those objects until they

113 Instruments used to cut tissue and to avoid bleeding.

literally fell apart.

When I traveled to the United States as a visiting professor, I realized that in every operation that I performed, a new needle tip, a new pencil, a new cable and a new cautery plate were used. Without reservation or hesitation, those wonderful, expensive, basically new objects, desperately needed in other places, were discarded at the end of the operation. Soon, I learned that after the operation, when everybody was distracted, I could very carefully take those articles from the garbage, put them in my pocket and take them back home. Once, a nurse in the operating room saw me and very quietly came close to me, "Are you interested in these used cables?" I whispered back that we desperately needed them in Mexico. She told me she would give me more and returned with a huge plastic bag full of all of the cables used that particular day in the entire hospital. I was a little embarrassed but very happy. I put all the cables in my baggage and went back to Mexico.

When I arrived at the airport in Mexico City, the customs agent opened my bags. The man in charge made a theatrical face of surprise, "Electronic articles, impossible to pass."

So, I got close to him. Perhaps he expected me to try to bribe him. "Sir, I am the chief of surgery of IMAN. Look at these cables. Some still have dry blood on them. These are articles that our hospital is going to reuse because of our lack of resources. I hope that your son does not need an emergency operation and you come to the hospital and we tell you that we do not have the necessary equipment to operate on him." He did not know what to answer and just signaled with his hand, indicating for me to pick up my things and pass.

As time went by, I became more creative and "accidentally contaminated" a few cables (rather than a single one) during my operation because I knew these articles would go into the garbage. At the end of the operation, I waited until everybody left the room and then I smuggled the cables in my pocket.

On one occasion, I visited one of the most important children's hospitals in the United States while there was a very prominent professor of pediatric surgery visiting from China. China was beginning to open up after many years of restriction from its communist rule. This was, possibly, the first professor of pediatric surgery to be granted permission to visit a western country. One could see by the way he dressed, how precarious the Chinese economy was: He bought six-dollar glasses at one of the US airports. The belt in his pants was made of a single size that could fit anybody in his country. His denture was not custom made; he had to go to a store in Beijing and try a number of dentures until he found one that was suitable. He happened to be a lovely person and maybe the most prominent and respected pediatric surgeon in all of China.

During the time of the Chinese Cultural Revolution, he was punished and fired from his job as chief and professor of pediatric surgery and was sentenced to clean the streets. The doctor was considered a revisionist and was punished because he had a piano, a typewriter and even a pediatric surgery book written in English by Dr. Robert Gross! To the Chinese government, all of these things were manifestations of a capitalistic ideology. Some of his students and other young members of the Cultural Revolution physically punished him. He went on like that for four years. After that time, the government deemed him "rehabilitated" and he was able to return to his work. Amazingly enough he did not sound particularly bitter about what he had endured.

The Chinese professor was very interested in watching my operation. I felt his presence during my entire procedure, looking over my shoulder. I managed to "contaminate" a few cables during that operation. When I finished, I looked in the garbage can for the cables but they were gone. Then I looked at the Chinese professor and noticed the cables in his pocket.

Necessity is the mother of invention.

A MEXICAN SINGER IN JAPAN

Every year, the Pacific Association of Pediatric Surgeons brings together pediatric surgeons from many countries of the Pacific Ocean. These meetings emphasize camaraderie and a relaxed atmosphere—it is perhaps the friendliest pediatric surgical organization going. Traditionally, there is a party during which everybody in attendance must sing a folk song from his native country. I've always enjoyed that event. At one such gathering, I had the pleasure of meeting many distinguished Japanese pediatric surgeons, which prompted the Japanese Association of Pediatric Surgeons to generously invite me to be guest speaker during one of its annual meetings in Tokyo.

About three months before the meeting, I received a letter from the Japanese Association of Pediatric Surgeons president, "Dr. Peña, we are aware that you like to sing. We would be delighted if you would be willing to do so during our final dinner."

I enthusiastically accepted the proposal and about a month later, I received another letter, "We are looking forward to meeting you in Japan. In order to prepare our program, we are requesting the title of the song that you will perform."

At this time, I stopped laughing and began to worry. Something that is taken lightly and casually in a country like Mexico, where everybody sings after a minor provocation, may not be the same in Japan. Here I was, a Mexican shower singer trying to decide what to sing in front of a group of Japanese pediatric surgeons known for their seriousness and formality. I tried to think of a Mexican song that is popular all over the world and decided that "Bésame Mucho" was the right choice.

Two months later I was in Tokyo. On the day of the banquet I was handed an official program: First, words by some of the distinguished senior members of the Japanese Association of

Pediatric Surgeons. Second, a string quartet performing *The Four Seasons* by Vivaldi. Third, "Bésame Mucho" composed by Consuelo Velázquez, as performed by Dr. Alberto Peña. I paled and rushed to the bar to drink two emergency sakes!

When my turn arrived, a large piano was brought into place on stage and a Japanese pianist, wearing an impeccable tuxedo, appeared. The music for "Bésame Mucho" was already at the piano and sure enough, I sang like I was in the shower at home.

When I finished, my Japanese colleagues applauded excitedly. So much so, that I decided to give them an encore. However, when I turned to tell the pianist the name of the song, he was no longer there! I am sure he felt that his reputation was at risk—he did not want to be a part of such destructive musical misadventure. So, I sang alone. Through the years, I've become convinced that the warm ovation of my Japanese friends was not a tribute to my musical talent but rather to my courage.

*****

Traveling affords the means to learn about the values, habits, religions, traditions and political systems of other human beings. In spite of these differences, it is remarkable to recognize the similarities among all human beings. For me, traveling represents the singular honor of establishing common ground with people all over the planet: the parents of a sick child, the local pediatric surgeons trying to learn more, the philanthropic organizations from various countries and governments joining me for the purpose of improving the quality of a child's life. It is like flying at a higher level, above prejudices and within ideological differences. Traveling is an illuminating experience.

TWO MAIN CONCERNS ABOUT THE NEW GENERATION OF SURGEONS

When I was about 40 years old, I had a conversation with my 75-year-old father. I was complaining about many problems that society must face: corruption, crime, overpopulation, social inequality, intolerance, discrimination, bigotry, environmental destruction and the list went on. My father smiled, "I think you are getting old, Alberto." He explained that society must have confidence in young generations to look at these problems with a fresh perspective and to have innovative and imaginative approaches to all of them, without being overwhelmed. There must be faith in humankind and evolution; otherwise, people will struggle with pessimistic negative attitudes—a philosophic position that does not benefit anybody and contributes wholly to unhappiness.

I am always impressed by the intelligence and creativity of

young medical students and doctors. It is always enjoyable to talk and share ideas with residents and students, hearing their thoughts about the challenges confronting the medical and surgical fields. A fresh, though frequently naïve, less prejudiced approach to professional problems is always welcomed and sometimes quite creative. In my mind, there is no question that the new generation of doctors is better suited than the old ones. This is a sincere conviction. Medical students have the opportunity to obtain more knowledge now than in previous generations. If I finished medical school today, I would have to study more and work harder to achieve my academic goals because I would be up against more serious competition from my colleagues.

In the last 100 years, medicine and surgery progressed more than in all history. Throughout my professional career, medicine and surgery advanced in ways that I never dreamt possible. It was only a few years back that anatomy was learned from artistic renditions—products of the imagination of medical illustrators. Medical students were supposed to memorize the names of structures that they could not see, that had questionable, functional and practical importance. During an anatomy final exam, a sadistic professor would ask students to describe a humerus while presenting a femur,[114] in order to intentionally confuse and fail them. I never imagined that physicians would eventually learn anatomy and make precise diagnoses while referencing images of tridimensional

114 Main bone of the upper arm and main bone of the thigh, respectively. Each bone resembles the other.

computer-reconstructed sections of a real human body (like the images obtained with MRI[115] and CAT scans[116] studies).

At the present time, medical students and future doctors represent the final product of a sophisticated process of selection that actually begins in elementary school and continues through high school and college. Most of the young doctors I am familiar with are extremely intelligent and knowledgeable. It is almost impossible these days, to find a young doctor who does not know the basic anatomic and/or physiologic facts of the human body. In spite of all the developments and progress, I still have two concerns related with the selection of the new generations of surgeons:
1) Technical Dexterity and the Mystery of Surgical Skill: Being able to distinguish between doctors who have the capacity to perform good surgical procedures and those who do not. 2) Dedication: Being able to predict how much intelligence and talent a young doctor is willing to devote to the welfare of the patient.

Technical Dexterity and the Mystery of Surgical Skill

A DISTINGUISHING CAPACITY

Throughout the world, medical and surgical organizations have been making efforts to select the best professionals to practice medicine and surgery. A series of filters were created to make it

115 Magnetic resonance imaging- Use of nuclear magnetic resonance to produce images of the molecules that make a substance, especially the soft tissues of the human body.

116 Computerized axial tomography- Imaging method in which a cross-sectional image of the structures in a body is reconstructed by a computer from x-rays projected through the body.

nearly impossible for a non-intelligent or non-knowledgeable individual to become a doctor; nevertheless, I am still apprehensive. I believe that there is not a creative enough mechanism to identify, early in the professional life, those doctors possessing the dexterity and skills to become good technical surgeons and separate them from those who do not. Being intelligent and knowledgeable does not mean a person is a good technical surgeon or a dedicated doctor. Technical limitations of an individual are usually detected near the end of their training, when it is seemingly too late to stop and advise them to change specialty. This introduces a controversial issue: Can anybody be trained to become an excellent technical surgeon? I believe that the answer to this is no and I recognize that many of my colleagues do not agree with my point of view.

It is probably true that any human being with an average IQ can be trained to do most of the surgical operations performed today. Some will perform these operations in a very smooth, neat, efficient and technically adequate way, whereas others will perform these same procedures in a rough, bloody, careless, inadequate way with an increased number of complications (morbidity). If that morbidity is not very significant, these surgeons may actually spend their entire career doing those kinds of operations without being legally restricted to practice, in spite of those professionals who are unfortunate enough to work with them, silently enduring their technical limitations.

In a hospital, the professionals who know the distinction

between bad and good technical surgeons are the scrub nurses, senior residents and some anesthesiologists. They whisper about the next operation that a unanimously recognized "bad surgeon" will perform. And they consider it a punishment to work with certain other surgeons. Despite knowing they are co-participants of surgical misadventures and "very difficult" operations, these professionals cannot refuse to participate with the "bad surgeons." I have had the good fortune and honor to operate in hospitals all over the world. When I was able to have confidential conversations with surgical residents and other members of the surgical team, they usually named surgeons considered to be excellent—the ones trusted enough to operate on a relative. And, as expected, they also listed a few surgeons they would never allow to operate on a relative.

In other words, within each hospital, there are two unofficial lists of surgeons: one list of "good surgeons" and another list of "bad surgeons." Since it is taboo to discuss this topic, those lists never become official. If I am visiting a city and suddenly need an operation, I do not just grab the phone book or ask for the president of the local surgical association or the chief of surgery to operate on me. Rather, I call a local personal friend who knows the surgical environment well enough to recommend who preferentially should do my operation and who definitely should not.

Still, the question remains: Is it possible to detect among young candidates, those who are going to be excellent technical surgeons from those who will not? Possibly, but I believe this has not been achieved at the present time. So, the current system for selecting and training young surgeons must be improved and those involved with educating young surgeons must keep trying to progress.

Unpleasantly, I have dealt with a young physician in the final phase of his surgical training (eight years after graduating med school) and all the members of a surgical staff who believed he should not practice because of his incapability. The surgeons in charge of the training program decided to send the young doctor to rotate through my service, under my supervision for a period of time. I later learned that they wanted to obtain an unbiased opinion about the doctor's surgical skills. After his rotation, I was convinced that this young doctor should not be a surgeon although he was particularly talented in other means. He could give lectures about sophisticated surgical and research subjects, all based in theory. He graduated from one of the most prestigious Ivy League medical schools, he was educated, sociable and intelligent; yet, at the end of a relatively simple surgical procedure, he made comments indicating that he was incapable of perceiving and understanding the basic steps of the operation. It was a considerably painful incident. What followed was a serious litigation problem and the young physician never practiced pediatric surgery.

That, of course, was an extreme instance of an incapacity to operate; however, there are many other cases in which individuals are not as appalling but are known to have trouble operating. And still, there is no way to detect these doctors early enough to avoid problems and re-orient them towards another specialty. Allowing these surgeons to continue is detrimental for their career, their patients and members of the entire profession. Many of them could achieve much more if they were willing to practice another specialty. They would most likely enjoy their work, be academically more successful and above all, they would not hurt patients. I also believe these surgeons contribute to worsen the litigating environment of the practice.

In an ideal world, staff members of a specific hospital should be able to prevent bad technical surgeons from practicing. Conceivably, this could decrease the participation of lawyers and administrators in making decisions that should be left up to surgical boards. Since it is not easy and is politically incorrect, no one has been brave enough to act upon this. Surgeons and other medical professionals can always whisper the names of those who should not operate but they are not willing to say it officially or to prevent them from doing so. This is a very controversial subject and I am aware that there is a great deal of subjectivity in deciding that an individual is incapable of operating. It must be terrible to be prohibited to operate because somebody "believes" that you do not operate well.

There are individuals, though, who manage to instill in everyone around them that they are "bad surgeons." Perhaps a special board of professionals within each institution could be assembled to discuss what should be done about the extreme cases of these unanimously condemned individuals. Proactively and early in their careers, young physicians should be prevented from becoming surgeons once they have clearly demonstrated they lack necessary skills. There should be good vocational advice and orientation provided to medical students as well, allowing them to recognize their own talents and limitations.

If the operation is difficult, you are not doing it properly.

Dr. Robert Gross had these words written on his operating room wall and after my training, I worked at another institution and wrote the same words on the operating room wall. Some surgeons liked it very much; others were irritated by it. Interestingly, those who disliked Dr. Gross's idea were generally considered not to be good surgeons by the majority of doctors and nurses in the operating room.

When surgeons attend surgical meetings, surgical techniques are reviewed but not surgical skills. It is understood that an operation can be done with varying standards of quality but surgeons insist upon comparing results of the operations as if they were done with a consistent level of quality. In an era of "evidence-based surgery,"[117] this creates serious doubts and may even invalidate some conclusions drawn from multi-institutional evaluations of a

117 Growing demand for physicians to find, assess and implement methods of diagnosis and treatment on the basis of the best available current research, their clinical expertise and the needs and preferences of the patient. See page 293 for further discussion.

surgical technique. No two operations are totally alike.

There are operations that are technically more demanding than others, particularly in unexpected emergency situations such as trauma. During these procedures, incidents and misadventures may occur. On the contrary, elective operations can be planned in advance and are repeated many times throughout a professional's career; therefore, it is possible to improve the technique to the point of doing it in a proficient and technically correct manner. I believe that in most of the planned elective operations there is neither place nor justification for complications. Through my professional life I interacted with many kinds of surgeons. Some of them were rough good surgeons possessing the good judgment to select a subspecialty requiring that kind of surgeon. Others were fine, meticulous surgeons performing beautiful delicate operations benefiting many patients. I also interacted with many definitely bad surgeons who harmed a lot of people. I even witnessed a good surgeon change into a bad one because of his age and his incapacity to appreciate the right time to retire. However, I never met a bad surgeon who became good. In fact, some of the bad surgeons that I met got worse when they got older and impatient. The question then becomes, how can future "bad" technical surgeons be detected early enough? Certainly not in the way it is attempted now.

Perhaps young surgeons, incapable of operating, could be detected if senior surgeons were allowed to work with them closely for an entire year before they are officially accepted into a surgical training program. Dedicating one year of a surgical career to the selection of the right individual sounds very expensive and complicated to implement but I firmly believe that it is worthwhile when trying to benefit patients, decrease surgical morbidity and make many physicians happy by redirecting their vocational path.

DEXTERITY, SKILL AND THE MIND'S EYE

There is something magical about surgical skills: the elements that are required for a surgeon to perform a technically efficient, adequate, smooth and elegant operation are not easily defined. What is it that makes a "good surgeon" as opposed to a "bad surgeon," even with identical training? Sometimes, a surgeon's technical skills are compared with the dexterity of musicians, particularly those who use their hands. Surgeons and musicians may be comparable to a point but there are many significant distinctions. Of course, not included in this analysis are complex factors related with the art of musicians such as feeling, inspiration and beauty. Everyday, a piano player exercises the movement of her fingers, looking at the composition and the keyboard, which is always static. The pianist practices so much that she may play the piano with her eyes closed, without reading the music or looking at the instrument. That is not possible in surgery.

Operating is like playing an instrument, except that the instrument is fluid, changing every minute. It is like being a piano player while altering the type of piano and composition from one moment to the next. In each operation, the patient is not the same, the circumstances are not the same, and in fact, they change constantly. During an operation, an uninterrupted stream of information from the operative field travels through the eyes and is processed in the brain, generating multiple questions, demanding quick decisions in order to continue successfully.

Undoubtedly, anatomic and functional limitations in the movements of the hands represent a serious restriction in the practice of surgery. There are surgeons who can move their fingers and hands in a very fast, coordinated and elegant way. Some are even good piano players, violin players or guitar players; however, they are not necessarily good surgeons.

When I visited Florence, Italy, I had the pleasure to contemplate and admire Michelangelo's famous wonderful statue *David*. I was reminded of Michelangelo's response after being congratulated for his magnificent sculpture. Michelangelo claimed that *David* was already there and all he had to do was to remove the extra stone to reveal him. Of course, I hope the reader finds humor in my translation, but the fact remains—during the dissection of structures in the human body, a surgeon requires a certain degree of imagination or, should I say, a realistic three-dimensional concept of what he is trying to do. Like the Renaissance artist, a surgeon's *David* should already be present.

A tumor is viewed in a MRI study: its position, as well as the important surrounding anatomic structures that could be damaged during an attempted resection, are noted. Then, the surgeon enters the operating room with a specific idea as to what should be done. The dissection is conducted and guided, in part, by the pre-conceived, spatial concept in the surgeon's mind. Some individuals, regardless of how intelligent or well trained they are, cannot acquire this.

INTRA-OPERATIVE DECISION-MAKING PROCESS

Surgeons like to say:

Not making a decision is worse than making a wrong decision.

In addition to the pure dexterity and oculomotor cycle[118] exerted by surgeons, there is another, very interesting phenomenon occurring in an operation that I call the "intra-operative decision-making process." Despite of the multiple attempts to standardize surgical techniques and create well-defined technical steps for every operation, it turns out that in every case, the surgeon confronts various changing scenarios and dilemmas. Because of this, the surgeon must be capable to recognize when to move quickly and more importantly, when to slow down to deal with unexpectedly risky conditions. Being in a hurry and incapable of slowing down when necessary represents a recipe for complications. Even in operations that the surgeon has performed many times, he may find unexpected variables without precedent. The surgeon must then take a new initiative or improvise a maneuver that he has never

118 Receiving information through the eyes, processing it in the brain and generating a specific movement in the hands.

tried before. This creates a degree of trepidation in the surgeon. He will finish the operation with that concern in mind and may not sleep well that night. This is something that must be accepted as part of a surgeon's life. Some can live like that, others cannot.

There appears to be an emotional component in this process, something related with the fear of causing harm. Surgeons are always afraid of injuring the patient and in fact, patients are sometimes unintentionally hurt. The problem is unique, because the surgeon is obligated to make intra-operative decisions with an important degree of uncertainty in that moment. The surgeon cannot afford to leave the OR in the middle of an operation to go to the library to research and organize an intra-operative round table to discuss the subject. In other non-surgical specialties, doctors have time to contemplate, speculate, discuss and review the literature, eventually making a decision based on facts and evidence. In the operating room, though, the surgeon must take immediate action and must take risks. He may be wrong but he must learn to assume full responsibility for his actions and continue working. The so-called "evidence-based surgery" may gradually change this scenario to a point but this drama will continue for years to come.

Highly intelligent, analytic individuals, for whom making quick life and death decisions comes with a great deal of dread, must seriously consider becoming internists. A highly organized individual who likes to plan and anticipate everything in life may feel greatly frustrated when a surgical emergency produces disorder in his organized routine. For such persons, a surgical career may be the wrong profession. Young, talented surgeons have been paralyzed in the middle of an operation while trying to make a crucial decision, so afraid of harming the patient that they cannot decide what to do. A surgeon's life is all about making decisions without being sure that it is the correct one, confronting the consequences of the decisions later.

This means that the art of surgery and being a good surgeon requires more than skilled hands. It requires the entire circle: knowledge of the of surgery, experiences of similar cases, perception of the constantly changing operative field, an accurate, preconceived, spatial idea of the procedure processed in the brain and the intellectual and emotional capacity to make quick decisions with a degree of uncertainty.

Dedication

A CONVINCING CONVICTION

Attitudes are more important than aptitudes.

—*Anonymous*

From the purely conceptual and intellectual point of view, the technical practice of surgery is, broadly speaking, a non-sophisticated discipline. Understanding what a gastrectomy[119] or a pull-through[120] is all about does not require a high level of mental activity—it does not take complex abstractions or thinking

119 Removal of the stomach.

120 Removal the rectum and part of the colon to replace it with a healthy portion of the bowel.

mechanisms. If the basic principles of a cholecystectomy[121] were explained to high school students, they would be able to grasp the basic idea and repeat it very well.

Therapeutic decisions in surgery are also relatively simple. One does not have to be a genius to understand when a patient needs an operation and why. This means that a person can be a reasonably good surgeon with an average IQ, although being intelligent, has its advantages. Ironically, not all intelligent practicing surgeons are as good as expected. Most doctors and surgeons are bright and very well informed but it is relatively common to observe that their patients do not benefit fully from their talents. Why is this?

It does not matter how much money you have.
What matters is how much you are willing to give.

My grandmother used to say this about life and I believe something similar happens with intellect. Somebody may be rich in knowledge, intelligence and creativity, but if he is not authentically and sincerely interested in the patient's welfare, he may not benefit the patient. Surgeons are supposed to serve and help patients rather than use them to fulfill other selfish ambitions. Can young surgeons, who have a sincere, authentic interest in the patients' welfare, be discerned from those who do not? The answer is, not completely.

121 Removal of a gall bladder.

Every year, groups of young doctors—all dressing in a very similar way, speaking elegantly and behaving like well-educated, respectful individuals—are welcomed through the interviewing process of candidates for surgical training programs. They come to the interview with a cliché type autobiography and a series of letters of recommendation that basically describe their scores in the multiple tests that they passed throughout medical school or their previous training. Many times it is discerned that experienced surgeons coached these students to work hard at building the right curriculum. Nowadays, these young doctors must follow an entire strategy just to be accepted into a surgical program or even more so into a pediatric surgical program. The strategy is frequently implemented early in their career. These young doctors, for instance, are induced to do research and write articles, frequently on sophisticated subjects and certainly with what I consider to be the wrong motivation.

Occasionally, letters of recommendation are received from people who specifically refer to their conviction that a candidate will be an excellent doctor. Again, I believe that the only way this could be distinguished is if physicians were allowed to work with that candidate for an entire year, watching them make everyday decisions, seeing them interact with the nurses, parents, patients, children, grandparents and even the doorman, witnessing their responses to stressful situations.

Individuals with emotional disturbances tend to be very

intelligent. It is disconcerting to see highly educated, well trained, academically oriented physicians with an impeccable curriculum, suffer from border line serious emotional disturbances that only become obvious when it is too late to stop. Some of these individuals practice surgery for many years; frequently, the only clue that there is a problem is that they repeatedly change working places. In every hospital they worked, people whispered about them, but nobody (person or institution) dared to denounce the problem because they were concerned about the legal implication. It was simply easier to let the troublemaker doctor continue.

COMPASSION AND SINCERE INTEREST

All physicians talk and write about being compassionate and sincerely interested in the benefit of the patient. However, I believe that a person cannot be taught to feel compassion. A person cannot decide to become sincerely compassionate tomorrow. Some people are compassionate and others are not, whether they like it or not. Some people are almost too compassionate to the point of interfering with their every day practice.

Man can do what he wants but he cannot control what he wants.

—Arthur Schopenhauer

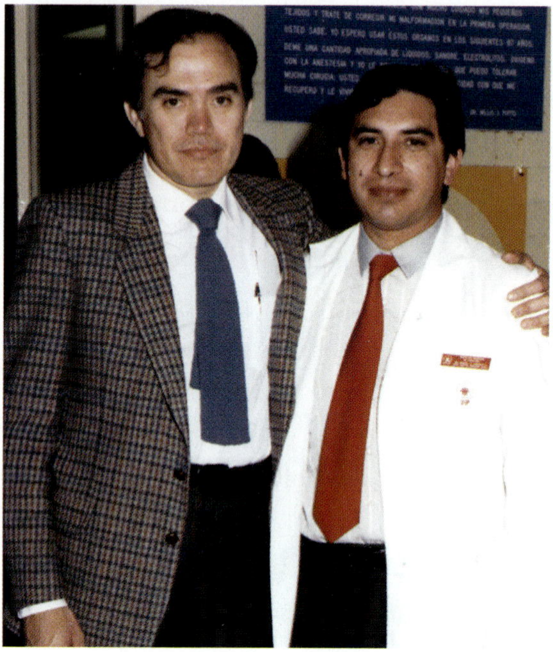

Alberto Peña and Miguel Vargas

I cannot forget an episode that occurred during my practice in Mexico City when I was working at the Central Military Hospital and INP. The distance between the hospitals is about 12.5 miles in a city with serious traffic problems. Miguel Vargas, chief resident at INP, was a sincerely dedicated young surgeon who eventually became a prominent pediatric surgeon in Mexico and with whom I always kept a good friendship. On this particular occasion, we were caring for an extremely sick child at INP. During the hours that I was working at the Central Military Hospital, I received frequent reports from Miguel and instructed him to implement measures to try to save the child's life. This went on for several days. At a critical time, I received a desperate call from Miguel. Things were not going well.

I left the Central Military Hospital in a rush and raced through the city. On my way toward INP, I was obsessively thinking about what could have gone wrong. I was ready to get to the bottom of the problem, to find all the possible mistakes and, if necessary, apply disciplinary actions.

Arriving at INP, I ran upstairs to the surgical floor. As I entered the room of the ill child, a nurse was covering his body. Miguel was at the end of the bed contemplating the scene; I could not see his face. I was upset and agitated and I asked many questions. When I walked toward the bed, I was able to see that Miguel's face was covered with tears. I stopped talking and tried to contain my own tears. It took numerous conversations with Miguel to convince him that he had done everything right. The kind of sensitivity and compassion that Miguel had was not acquired; it was something that was part of him.

It seems as though this is a main concern for those talented but uncompassionate individuals, for whom taking care of patients is not a goal but a way to achieve personal prosperity. Being able to detect compassionate, sincerely interested individuals (like Miguel) early in their careers is certainly not easy, but it is also not impossible. I do not believe that simple written tests, evaluations, multiple publications, sophisticated planned research activities, an Ivy League education, participation in Boy Scout activities or religious oriented missions necessarily guarantee that a doctor will use his intellect to fully benefit the patient. Once more, I believe that only closely working together on a daily basis and observing the behavior of a potential candidate, under various circumstances, may present a fair idea of their positive and negative aspects.

Many doctors like to talk about the practice of medicine and surgery as a kind of philanthropic activity that requires sacrifice and torture. I disagree. If doctors like what they do, they have more chances to do a better job and exercise their creativity. Those young candidates who are willing to suffer and be tortured should not be pursued; instead, candidates who love practicing surgery and believe it is a privilege to work long hours, doing what they enjoy, should be considered. This search should appraise those candidates who can sincerely say, like my father Federico:

I always did what I liked the most and I even got paid for doing it!

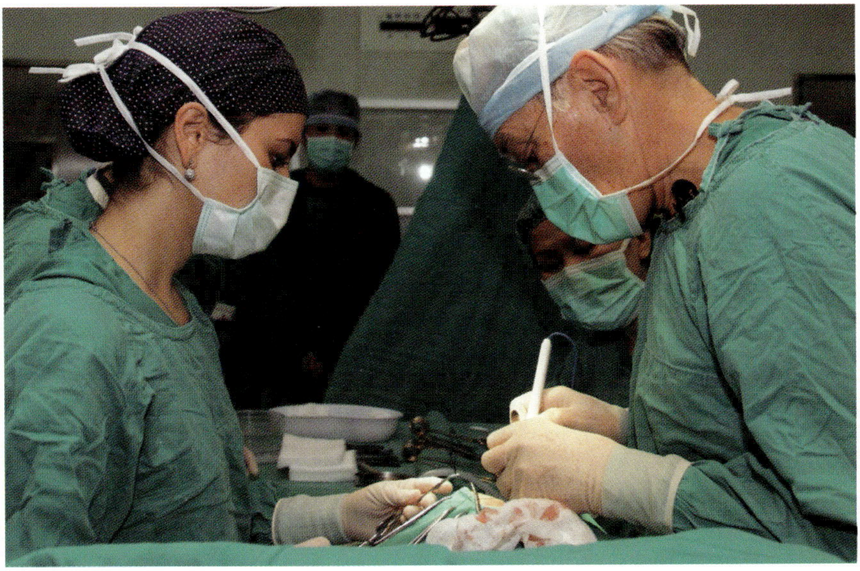

THE SURGICAL TEAM

To perform a technically sound operation, adequate support is required. Surgeons are responsible for the assistants collaborating with them. If a surgeon works with an extremely skilled and knowledgeable assistant, the operation becomes easier and the assistant becomes a very active member of the team. Frequently, though, surgeons do not select surgical assistants and the operation is conducted with an unfamiliar, non-experienced or awkward aide. Since surgeons are responsible for the final outcome of the operation, strategies must be implemented to employ the assistant's skills or to neutralize a dangerous assistant.

An extremely important member of the surgical team is the scrub nurse or scrub technician. The importance of this person cannot be overemphasized. In an ideal world, the scrub nurse should master the art of anticipation—an indispensable characteristic of that profession. For that, the scrub nurse must constantly be aware of the operative field. It is integral for them to be familiar with the technique and the particular way a surgeon operates. To achieve that, it is necessary for the surgeon to have, as much as possible, a systematic, disciplined, methodic way of operating.

Good scrub nurses struggle when operating with a surgeon who does not use a systematic approach or when other surgical assistants are situated between them and the surgeon. As a consequence, the scrub nurse's view of the operative field is blocked and they are unable to predict and anticipate the surgeon's needs. Chaos ensues: a screaming surgeon complains because he does not get the right instrument at the right time and a scrub nurse is intimidated, praying for an end to the distress of a bloody surgical misadventure.

Scrub nurses can also be divided into bad and good ones. Most bad scrub nurses never become good. The reason may be that they do not really like the profession or they simply lack the habit of looking into the operative field to understand what is happening. Dispassionate, slow, bitter, negative scrub nurses waiting for the verbal order to deliver every single stitch or instrument are a burden. They must be dragged through several hours, increasing the operative time and making others (including the patient) suffer with them. A scrub nurse's proficiency is not necessarily related with IQ or degree of knowledge. The person may be very intelligent and may possess a master's degree but if uninterested, they are not going to be an efficient team member. A dynamic, attentive, anticipating, interested, optimistic scrub nurse is the most valuable figure of the surgical team. Together, surgeon and scrub nurse, working repeatedly in elective procedures, may reach a high degree of efficiency—the operation runs smoothly, elegantly, quickly and enjoyably. It is akin to a concert and the interaction between the director and musician. This is how excellence can be achieved during the performance of an operation. Excellence is what all surgeons must try to attain. Excellence is what patients and their parents expect.

As time goes by, hospitals and operating rooms grow in number, size and technical complexity. Admittedly, the administrations of those facilities are extremely complicated and that may be why surgeons have been losing more and more power to designate their own assistants. It is extremely difficult for administrators and head nurses of the operating rooms to please a surgeon and designate the scrub nurse considered optimally competent for a specific operation. It is unfortunate that a surgeon must sometimes try to perform a rather complex and lengthy operation with a sub-optimally trained or an experienced scrub nurse, unconcerned about the surgical act and insensitive to surgeon's needs. If a surgeon asks for a specific scrub nurse to work with exclusively, to reach that high degree of coordination, it is frequently considered a prima donna type of request.

Understandably, administrators prefer to deal with interchangeable professionals with consistently good standards of quality. It is enormously complicated to work and organize big conglomerates of surgeons and scrub nurses, accepting that there are excellent ones, good ones, average ones and bad ones. The whole concept is non-manageable from the administrative point of view. The reality is that there are various, varying capabilities of surgeons and scrub nurses, even though their credentials do not reflect this. All human beings alike accept and aim for excellence, in every kind of human activity, particularly in dealing with a surgical procedure. Excellence does not occur in a widespread way. So, surgeons and members of the surgical team can only try to achieve it at a personal level.

CHARGING THE EMOTIONAL BATTERIES

During my professional life, particularly during my training, I was privileged to have access to highly reputed institutions. I interacted with very talented colleagues and was frequently impressed by their creativity and vast knowledge. A number of them became brilliant, famous surgeons to the advantage of many patients. But not all of them achieved what I expected. The explanation for this usually resided in non-professional factors: emotional disturbances, family problems, unfulfilled expectations, anxieties, dissatisfaction with surgery due to lack of vocation and extenuating working hours. And all of these factors frequently resulted in a rather unhealthy lifestyle.

It is obvious that emotions are not always controlled by intellect and this may be why many intelligent individuals have the inability to achieve their goals. Some of my highly competitive colleagues came from highly competitive families. Since they were little children they were indoctrinated; not only did their parents expect great things from them but these individuals also had very high expectations for themselves. As a consequence, they were programmed to be extremely ambitious and to achieve high goals. As time went by, though, they confronted reality in its various forms.

Extremely intelligent surgeons may find it easy to solve most of the academic, administrative and political problems confronted throughout their careers. Nevertheless, the art of surgery, as a purely technical act, may not come as easily. A relatively simple operation may become a humbling experience and can be a serious source of frustration, irritating the highly sophisticated, intellectual, academic surgeon, particularly if they do not enjoy it or do not possess the necessary characteristics to be good surgeons.

Never underestimate a surgical procedure.

Nobody can claim to have ever mastered the art of surgery. Everyday, there is a possibility for a busy clinical surgeon to confront adversity. These trying events occur to every surgeon, regardless of intelligence, academic rank, number of research projects, grants, publications or authored books.

Sometimes, ambition and high personal expectations provoke a surgeon to impose an unattainable discipline on their everyday life, affecting their health. A very competitive individual, for instance, might consider it a waste of time to sleep. They do not respect their body: they have long working hours, they overeat, abuse coffee and sometimes alcohol or even drugs. Personal problems at home also add to the very serious distractions interfering with their practice.

Confronting problems in the hospital requires a fresh, emotionally stable mind and a capacity to concentrate without interruption. It is impossible for someone to do that if they have serious emotional disturbances or troubles at home. It is extremely important to have a healthy personal life in order to be successful. For this, I encourage young surgeons to define their priorities and remember that the patient's welfare is the center of a physician's world.

Ideally, a surgeon must find enough pleasure and satisfaction in his everyday practice to be able to go home without taking any professional problems with him. By the same token, he is supposed to "charge his emotional batteries" at home to avoid letting his personal troubles and concerns interfere with his professional activity. Varying from one person to the other, "charging the emotional batteries" refers to non-professional activities and diversions that give pleasure and fulfill emotional and cultural needs. A successful marriage, love, family, playing sports, hobbies and living a healthy life are just a few things to enjoy.

*****

Practicing surgery in order to publish, accumulate cases, make more money and compete to obtain higher academic ranks represents spurious motivations. Surgery must be enjoyed; surgeons must focus on doing tomorrow's case better. By doing so, other rewards (academic, economic, etc.) come in due time. Although the real, true reward in a surgeon's life must come from a patient's successful recovery and the never-ending desire to improve upon the next operation. In other words, I suggest to all surgeons:

Do your best and leave the rest to the gods.

A medical student, who has been the best of his class, becomes the best resident of his generation and eventually a young attending surgeon. He is a perfectionist and has extremely high standards. He not only expects the institution that he works for to be perfect, but the university, the city, the country and perhaps the world. But this is an imperfect world; inefficiency is everywhere. And there is the unavoidable human factor. Human beings represent a spectrum that spans from extremely talented to not so talented, from very efficient, to efficient, to inefficient and to very inefficient.

Daily, a surgeon walks into a hospital and finds that things were not done exactly to their specifications and their patients do not always recover the way that was expected. The surgeon must be calm and think about the problems, devising realistic, feasible solutions, not expecting that the next day everything will be perfect.

In medicine, a surgeon must depend on a large series of individuals to collaborate with them—people with varying respectable views, priorities, talents and opinions, frequently different from their own. A surgeon must learn to take the best from each of them.

Expecting high performance in every human being sometimes produces the opposite effect. Pushing individuals to try to get too much from them, beyond their capacity, may produce similar negative returns. Physicians must recognize that things cannot always be the way they like. Some perfectionists have temper tantrums whenever they find things are not working the way they expected, making them angry. Angry people aggravate those who work around them, creating a tense working environment. Having no harmony in the work place is almost a tragedy because surgeons spend more time in the hospital than at home awake. If they are not happy at work, they are going to be eternally frustrated.

It is not easy to learn and accept the distinction between what is ideal and what is real and plausible. The words "ideal" and "idealistic" are used when referring to dreams, fantasies and levels of wanton success but they also belong to the world of ideas that people work everyday to try to make reality. Fantasies, dreams and ideals sometimes become real which makes people very happy. Sometimes it is impossible to make a reality out of fantasy, which of course is not pleasant, but should never be a source of extreme frustration. Life and profession is always a confrontation between ideals and reality.

Surgeons should go to work every day knowing that they are going to confront new and unexpected types of problems, understanding that they are paid to solve them. Expecting to find that everything in the hospital has been done according to their instructions and the patients have excellent postoperative course because they performed what was thought to be a perfect operation, may not be always true.

When visiting a hospital, people only see the friendly aspects of it; they cannot appreciate, as visitors, the problems that exist in all organizations of human beings, including politics, egos, unfair competition and so on. It is not uncommon for a surgeon to believe that his hospital is full of problems. This may be followed by the fantasy that other medical institutions are much better. The result is, frequently, a surgeon who constantly changes jobs, searching for the ideal institution that is free of problems but does not exist. He focuses on the hospital and all of the professionals working there as the main source of his frustration.

The main challenge and enemy to beat is inside of us.

Frustration causes individuals to complain. And complaining and moaning does not benefit anybody. In fact, human beings stray away from those people. I grew up in a developing country where doctors had many reasons to criticize and complain: underdevelopment, the lack of funds to practice good medicine, the lack of material and equipment, the lack of resources to do research, the lack of stimuli to have a decent academic life, I could go on and on.... In those countries, frequently, it is believed that in the so-called "developed" world, these problems do not exist. To my surprise, when I moved to the United States, the most technically and medically advanced country in the world, I found that doctors there also complained! In a way, I think they sometimes complained even more. It almost seems like humans are a critical and reproachful species. Occasionally, I meet people who never complain. I wonder what their secret is.

I suggest that young surgeons try to stay away from cynical and pessimistic individuals. I also believe in trying to keep medical students and residents away from negative, pessimistic mentors and professors. Some of these negative surgeons recommend to their own children that they not become surgeons. That shows how much they suffer in their own profession.

Very ambitious, talented, young surgeons that are well informed may think they have the answer for problems in the department of surgery; they feel that they have the talent and capacity to advise the chief of surgery what to do. Also, they think that they know how to run the hospital, the city and even the country! Yet, real problems are usually right in front of them. In the specific case of surgeons, their job consists of avoiding complications and performing better and better operations everyday. By doing so, surgeons have accomplished their task and do not have to worry so much about the problems of the world. In theory, a surgeon could reach a point in his career in which he could say that he performs impeccable operations followed by no complications. Until then (and if he has extra time), he could start proposing solutions for the hospital, for the city and for the country. In reality, that never happens.

An entire life is not enough to master the art of surgery.

DISTRACTORS

In surgery, like in all other professions, there are distractors—activities or troubles that deviate surgeons' minds away from their primary task. If one sits in a surgeons lounge and listens to some of the conversations, it is amazing the number of subjects that are discussed. What is more impressive to perceive is that some surgeons appear to be more concerned about other things rather than their performance. As all humans, surgeons may suffer from excessive ambition, inter-departmental struggles, monetary issues, jealousy, unfair competition, envy and egos incompatibility; still, they must make an effort to avoid these predicaments so not to divert too much mental energy needed to improve patients' welfare.

MONEY

Money, of course, is extremely important because of its great influence upon modern society—people cannot live without it. Money is probably one of the most common distractors for surgeons. It is perfectly legitimate for a surgeon to try to obtain enough resources to guarantee a decent living for himself and his dependents. The quandary is that sometimes the concern about money grows well beyond those basic needs. There is something disturbing about seeing a surgeon in between operations call his stockbroker or to overhear a physician worried about his yacht or other businesses. All of this is legal; however, one would expect a surgeon to be so focused on the operation that he just finished or the next one scheduled that he would not have time to devote to playing the market.

The concern about money, of course, may be more or less serious in different countries. In some countries, money is a real and legitimate worry. There are countries where the government and political system determine a doctor's salary to be equivalent to the humblest peasant, countries where the doctors do not have enough money to even buy a pair of shoes. Surprisingly, these doctors do not necessarily complain more than the doctors in the rich countries! In some developing countries, the doctors' salaries are extremely low and it makes sense to hear that doctors struggle to get more compensation. Some doctors must have multiple jobs in various institutions or combine the practice of a government hospital with a private practice in order to take home enough money to fulfill their basic needs. In most of the countries that I visited, though, I did not see what one could call a really poor doctor, meaning, somebody who had no money to eat or to feed their family.

It is one thing for doctors to be concerned about survival and fulfilling their needs and it is completely another for them to be preoccupied to a point in which their talents are not used for their patients. Instead, they become overwhelmed by economic and business strategies, investment methodology, reimbursement strategies, market share, administration of the practice, insurance, HMOs,[122] coding strategies and all the sophisticated modern ways to obtain money in the practice of medicine.

ACADEMICISM

Physicians are expected to contribute to the advancement of science and technology. Originally and ideally, if one physician finds a better way to treat or cure a disease or obtains a better result with a specific new operation or treatment, they are supposed to determine the quickest and easiest way to communicate that to as many colleagues as possible, for the benefit of all patients. This is supposed to be the legitimate and authentic origin of academicism, as well as the reason to present papers and publish articles and books. Ironically, academicism is another distractor for surgeons.

Through the years, academic motivations have changed and become an extremely sophisticated series of activities that together I call pseudo-academicism. A modern consequence of all this is that some institutions, particularly those affiliated with universities and university hospitals, expect a certain "level of productivity"

122 Health maintenance organization- Corporation that is financed by insurance premiums and has member physicians and professional staff who provide curative and preventive medicine within certain financial, geographic and professional limits to enrolled volunteer members and their families.

from their doctors to be consistent with the academic ranks that they hold. This, as expected, puts significant pressure on doctors to achieve a certain degree of "productivity" in order to be promoted. The consequence of which can be both positive and negative.

Yes, there are many exceptionally good articles and books to read but there are also an increasing number of publications that are basically copies and reproductions. There are even publications that simply present useless material. Being creative, learning from experience, creating new procedures and therapeutic methods are all welcome and should be shared with other colleagues in the form of publications; nevertheless, physicians should be very careful not to invert their priorities, reaching the point in which the urge to publish compromises the quality and authenticity of the publication. The number of publications a doctor has does not always represent the quality of care that a specific doctor delivers. Some authors of surgical textbooks and hundreds of articles are excellent surgeons, while others are not. I know brilliant, dedicated surgeons that I would trust to operate on anyone and they have never published a paper.

POLITICKING AND ADMINISTRATION

Politics and administrative aspirations represent two frequent distractors occupying the mind and time of many surgeons. Perhaps a better term for politics should be politicking, not only in national or city politics, but also within the hospital or specific department.

Administrators used to work diligently to facilitate the surgeon's performance in the operating room, in the clinic and in the patients' wards. Today, there is a tendency to make doctors and surgeons co-responsible for administrative issues. This is a very significant burden, as well as a time consuming activity, particularly for surgeons who are also chiefs. Still, someone has to manage the hospital. The higher a surgeon is in the hierarchy of the surgical pyramid, the more administrative obligations the surgeon will have. Some surgeons enjoy it very much, which is great for all the other doctors (like me) who enjoy practicing surgery. There is nothing better than having a good chief to tend to all the administrative issues, allowing surgeons to work comfortably and be dedicated full time to their practice.

Some surgeons are concerned because they want to escalate within the pyramid of hierarchy and become chiefs. I have witnessed excellent surgeons gain a reputation as being great mentors, operators, researchers and clinicians. They inspired generations of surgeons by contributing to the training of many young surgeons and benefiting thousands of patients. In spite of all that, they are unhappy because they have never been chiefs! Some eventually become chiefs, only to find that their professional life is nearly ruined. I have seen great surgeons become chiefs only to be fired or resign a few months later, not because of technical or academic incapacities but due to administrative problems. If that happens relatively soon after they become chiefs, it is possible for them to resume their original surgical activity. Some never really recover, which is quite sad.

Dr. Judah Folkman, chief of surgery at Children's Hospital Boston when I was in training, used to say:

Being chief of surgery is like being the director of an opera house, constantly dealing with prima donnas.

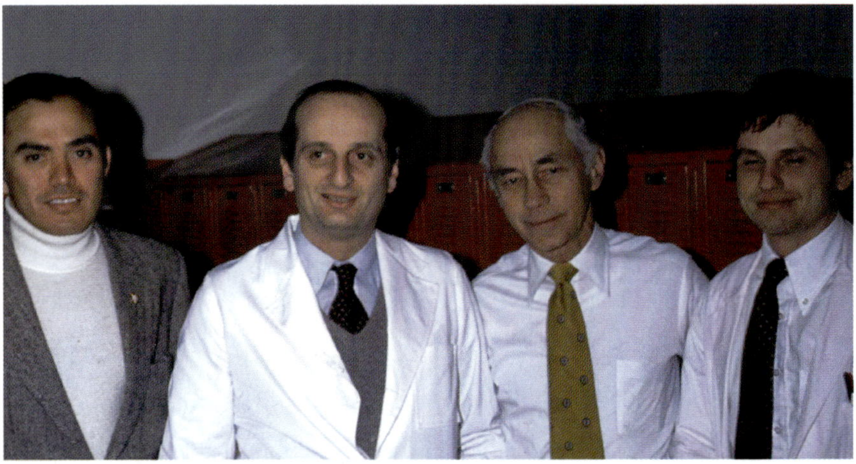

Left to right: Alberto Peña, Judah Folkman, Arnold Colodny, and Jay Vacanti

*****

There is a certain fantasy about being chief. Frequently, those who have not been chief do not understand the pressures and responsibilities that position carries. Being chief means to take upon a very heavy administrative burden for which special and alternate training is needed. From the moment a surgeon becomes a chief, he is not only responsible for the care of his patients but the care of all the patients of all the surgeons in his department. It is a skill and takes a special disposition to deal with the temperaments of other surgeons. Some surgeons have a particular talent making them very good administrators; they are very beneficial for the rest of the surgical community. Basically, they partially sacrifice their own clinical performance in order to create an adequate working environment for the other surgeons.

The only thing worse than being
an administrator is to be administered.

This concept is half true and it is frequently used as a rationalization to climb the hierarchic pyramid. Therefore, it is integral for a young surgeon to define as early as possible in his career, his goals as a clinical surgeon, investigator and administrator. The young surgeon should determine the amount of effort and time that he is willing to invest in each of these areas. If, for example, he decides that his passion is to care for patients, he must then look for an institution with a good chief, in an adequate environment, allowing him to do so. Before being trapped in the fantasy of becoming chief, the young surgeon should think about how much training, vocation and interest he has for politicking and administration.

LITIGATION

There is always a risk of being sued—litigation and medical legal problems are other very significant distractors in the practice of surgery. Physicians should learn about the most common factors predisposing them to a legal medical problem. Surgeons must be careful not to reach the point of inverting their priorities and end up practicing "defensive surgery." Surgeons cannot afford to employ so much of their mental energy trying to avoid litigation that they are diverted from their patients.

When traveling in a plane across the ocean, there is risk involved. When boarding the plane and offered a drink, it is assumed that the captain knows what to do. It would be very uncomfortable, upon entering the plane, to be welcomed by a lawyer with a document in hand and witness nearby, asking for a signed consent so the airline could avoid legal responsibility in case of a crash, a kidnapping or any other adverse event.

Informing the patient and their parents about their condition and the operation is a very important part of this practice. Unfortunately, it is also a legal obligation. This is unfortunate because doctors should already keep patients and parents well informed. A legal obligation implicitly means that there is a need for supervising and punishing those who do not do it. Is there a need for lawyers and police to remind physicians about their basic duties?

I do not believe doctors should provide unsolicited, irrelevant information solely to protect themselves and their institutions. The so-called "informed consent"[123] and the details given to parents sometimes reach the absurd. Continuing in that direction, surgeons will end up requesting consent for the type of suture that will be used. In fact, surgeons already do many things to patients in the OR without any consent. They perform many unexpected surgical maneuvers based on every minute changing operative circumstance, performing things that were not mentioned in the so-called "informed consent."

Here is a paragraph that I took directly from the operative report of a real medical record of a patient referred to me from another institution:

> *Prior to the procedure, I had a detailed conversation with the family regarding the risks, benefits and alternatives to the procedure. Specifically, I described what we were going to do and how it would likely benefit the patient. We talked about the surgical team and the fact that I would be assisted during the procedure by other physicians and nurses. We discussed my specific experience with this sort of procedure. I further informed the family about alternatives to surgery and the risks associated with not treating surgically or waiting to treat surgically. I was clear that there are risks with any procedure, including this one, and that it was possible that the procedure would not work. We talked about the potential need for additional surgery.*

123 Agreement by a patient for a surgical or medical procedure or participation in a clinical study after achieving an understanding of the relevant medical facts and the risks involved.

I described some of the possible complications and the relative likelihood of those complications. We specifically discussed the risks of infection, bleeding, postoperative pain, and even major complications such as paralysis, loss of major body function or death. Finally, I offered to the family the opportunity to repeat back their understanding and ask questions.

*****

The administrators of any hospital would be proud of this legally defensive, technically impeccable, cliché-type introduction of an operative report. The surgeon covered virtually all of the potential sources of complications. The irony is that this surgeon unsuccessfully performed the same operation, three times on the same patient! The patient had serious complications in all three procedures. In this case, the patient would benefit greatly by being referred to a surgeon with more experience in that particular operation; however, the surgeon persisted in trying to do the operation again for the fourth time. He asked the parents to sign an "informed consent," warning them about the possibility of even more complications not even included in the report. With these actions, it is visible that the surgeon's main objective is to avoid all responsibility; he is focused more on the potential legal implications of the operation instead of the welfare of the patient!

The "informed consent" is an unavoidable exercise in most

countries at the present time. Personally, I believe that parents understand that an operation is something serious for their child. There is something unpleasant about sitting in front of a patient or their mother and asking them to sign a legal document in order to perform an operation. It is impossible to avoid feeling like the stereotypical lawyer or a car dealer. Taken to an extreme, the "informed consent" could be translated as: "I am not responsible for what happens to the patient as a consequence of my operation." More and more the "informed consent" includes more and more possibilities of complications. Some consents, which I have read for the repair of something as simple as a hernia, include potential complications as remote as hemorrhage or death! In my entire career, I do not remember a hemorrhage or a death occurring during a hernia operation in a baby.

Some surgeons, like the one with the operative report referenced above, take special courses to learn exactly what to write in the medical record (a defensive legal jargon, what to say, what not to say), geared to succeed in the event of being sued. What ever happened to trying to be better surgeons? Using mental energy to write and talk in a legally and bureaucratically "correct way" is an inversion of priorities. A better way to prevent medical legal problems, I believe, is to be meticulous, scrupulous and dedicated to do better operations and to establish an authentic, respectful doctor-patient relationship. Many patients have adverse or unpredictably bad results from an operation, which is painful for everyone involved. Instead of being angry, defensive or too preoccupied about a potential legal suit, the best basic strategy must be to try to remain as close as possible to the patient and their parents, showing true concern about the patient's condition while earnestly trying to think about how to solve the problem. Rightfully so, the family is upset about the complication but they are much more upset by the surgeon's defensive attitude, lack of sincerity and dishonesty, refusing to accept responsibility and his conspicuous absence during the most trying moments. If a surgeon normally visits a postoperative patient everyday, in the event of an adverse postoperative course, it is highly desirable to see that patient several more times in a day. Not to just leave it to the "informed consent."

I know that it is probably too late to reverse this phenomenon because of all the complications patients have undergone in the past and the fact that doctors gradually (and perhaps unintentionally) allowed lawyers and bureaucrats to encroach upon activities that used to be based on good faith and confidence. Now doctors have to be compliant and work through this legal and bureaucratic process. I am extremely fortunate to have never been sued. I understand that I have been lucky and that it can happen to anybody but I believe there are certain important aspects of the doctor-patient relationship that help to avoid medical legal problems. Rather than putting an emphasis on the details and technicalities of the "informed consent," surgeons should never forget the primary and best way to fight this problem: avoid complications altogether and show patients or their parents a genuine interest and concern about the problem. This will, no doubt, develop a relationship based on respect, good faith and confidence rather than on a legal contract. Surgeons should also concentrate their mental energies on upcoming operations to avoid complications and to improve their everyday performance. I believe that by doing so, surgeons can better fight the litigation environment instead of creating more "efficient, technically correct, legally oriented, informed consent documents."

Law is a discipline of adversarial relationships.

—James P. Weaver, MD

I would like to add to Dr. Weaver's assertion by stating that medicine and surgery should be a discipline of the harmonious kind. I vividly recall a case in which a little baby that I operated on had a respiratory arrest in the middle of the night. The nurse in charge did not detect it early enough and the baby suffered brain damage. The family was a member of a prominent law firm and, as expected, they sued the hospital. Interestingly, they were kind enough to keep me away from the whole legal process. I never received a phone call from a lawyer. I did not even learn about this problem until years later. Surgeon-patient-family relationships must be based on the authentic and sincere concern from the surgeon and the faith, trust and cooperation from the family. This is the most valuable mechanism to avoid medical legal problems.

One of my professors from Mexico, Dr. Leonel Villavicencio, participated in a round table at the American College of Surgeons discussing medical legal issues. The surgeons were complaining about the growing litigation problem in the United States and they asked him how things were in Mexico. He replied, "We do not have those kinds of problems. In Mexico, when the patients get upset, they shoot at the surgeon!" Unfortunately, this was frequently true. I know of several cases in which doctors were killed.

It is not pleasant for surgeons to see that some patients or their relatives sue a doctor without real justification and how many times the predicament is exacerbated by unscrupulous lawyers. On the other hand, there are countries where a humble patient can never contemplate suing a prominent doctor in spite of being a victim of obvious malpractice. I have been in places where the doctors clearly perform malpractice, they are aware of what they are doing, they are cheating the patients and sadly, the corrupted legal system does nothing to protect the patients. With all the negative aspects and inconveniences of the increasing litigating atmosphere in the United States, it is necessary to put things in perspective and remember that everything is relative.

The patients or their parents do not know much about medicine, but they have three very important characteristics: intuition, common sense and an authentic interest in healing. They know when a doctor is genuinely interested in the patient. They get upset when somebody lies to them, hides things from them and when they detect a lack of seriousness and respect.

I believe there should be more emphasis in selecting future surgeons who are legitimately concerned about their patients in lieu of training them more and more in the legal aspects of the practice of surgery. Practicing defensive medicine or surgery is a very unfortunate result of predicaments that surgeons should have confronted and prevented a long time ago. This probably happened because some surgeons did not behave in an ethically correct manner. Since then, surgeons have basically stepped down from the privileged position that society originally granted them, allowing the public to lose the confidence and trust in them that they once enjoyed.

BEING IN A HURRY

It is not good to be in a hurry,
particularly if you are on the wrong road.

Because of the surgeons' type of work, it is extremely common to see them in a constant hurry. Besides having most of the obligations that all physicians have—including caring for patients from the medical point of view, reading the recent literature to maintain a degree of expertise in the field, plus all the bureaucratic burdens that seem to be increasing nowadays—a large portion of a surgeon's time is spent operating. Surgery is an art that requires repetition and exposure to various kinds of scenarios and anatomic situations to be successful. Professional, first-class violin players practice as much as six to eight hours every day to maintain their skills. Something similar can be said about surgery. It is particularly risky and inadequate to be an "occasional surgeon." Surgery is unforgiving. If a surgeon abandons the repetition of the art of surgery and does not practice it enough, very soon, patient and doctor will feel the consequences.

There is no replacement for experience in the practice of good surgery—the surgical act itself takes an enormous amount of time and as a result, surgeons are often left with a very limited time to perform all of their other tasks. After a surgeon finishes in the operating room, he returns to his office to find many messages, unanswered phone calls, unanswered letters, imminent deadlines to write papers and many newly published papers that he is supposed to read. It all keeps piling up! He sits down to it all and it is already the end of the day. The product is a professional who is always in a rush. This is dangerous. Being in a hurry represents a risk of missing important facts and information that may result in the mistreatment of a patient. Being in a hurry does not allow the surgeon to enjoy the practice of surgery and may, I believe, interfere with the magnificent process of creativity.

During intermissions and coffee breaks of surgical meetings, surgeons' conversations frequently gravitate toward a popular subject: how "busy" a specific surgeon is. Not being "busy enough" is considered a defect representing a serious hindrance and something to gossip about. Surgeons like to boast, "Last year, I operated on 1000 cases." Supposedly, that is something to flaunt but nobody ever questions: Did you enjoy those cases? What did you learn from them? Are you satisfied with the results? Did you perform the operations with the same quality you would expect for your own child? Did you improve your technique as you gained more experience?

There is a very healthy routine that should be followed that I learned from a famous surgeon. After an operation is completed, a surgeon should spend five minutes alone to contemplate what happened during the procedure. "If I have to do this operation again tomorrow, what am I going to do to improve it?" All operations can be improved and upon reflection, there is always something that a surgeon is unhappy about. There is one part of the operation they did not like; there was a time in which they were uncomfortable. The exposure was not adequate, the light was not good and the surgeon was in a rush, finishing with an unpleasant feeling that cannot be verbalized.

First of all, if something is not going the way a surgeon likes or things are uncomfortable, he should pause and consider what is happening. The surgeon should think about his situation, the position of the patient, the exposure, the placement of the retractors, the position of the assistant, excessive noise, distracting frivolous conversations, extra-professional problems occupying his mind and anything else that might be taking away from the operation. Are the basic surgical principles being violated? Is the quality of the procedure being compromised because things are moving too hastily? Usually, there is a "yes" for one or several of these questions.

Sometimes an operation is booked with a preconception that it will be a simple, quick case, only to find that the opposite is true. The patient's anatomy turned out to be unexpectedly complex and the maneuvers necessary to repair the malformation were technically more demanding and time-consuming than first thought. Repairing a defect demands full focused attention, a delicate, meticulous technique and most importantly, it requires time. An unpleasant event frequently occurs on a day with a busy schedule, when everyone is mentally and emotionally prepared for quick and easy procedures, having many other ambitious activities planned for the day. This scenario is a recipe for a surgical misadventure. Under these circumstances, surgeons should use their mental energy to do the best possible job, making the necessary arrangements to cancel or re-book commitments and appointments outside the hospital, in the office or in the clinic.

*****

Official operative reports are usually dictated very quickly. Many reports are descriptions of impeccable surgical techniques that read as if they were taken from a surgery textbook. Coincidentally, some surgeons have a template saved on their computer to use for every operation they perform. Yet, the real operation is frequently full of undesirable incidents, forceful awkward maneuvers and unpleasant moments of hesitation, questionable technical maneuvers and unexpected findings, forcing improvised actions with uncertain effects. These events are generally not described in the official operative report, though, through a lifetime, they are the epitome of the real process of training for a surgeon.

In a surgeon's practice, they care for many patients that endured attempted, failed operative procedures or catastrophic surgical events that produced significant and otherwise preventable sequelae. When the surgeon reads the operative report of one of those operations, it often looks as if it was perfectly executed. What is uncovered during the re-operation is something completely contradictory. Something went wrong in the original operation—the faulty surgeon was not honest and did not take the time to record it in his report.

Another important, recommended routine is for surgeons to keep a diary of operations. A diary could represent a place to express doubts and insecurities. There are uncertainties in almost every operation and surgeons are encouraged to record them. During the patient's follow-up, they will learn if the operation was correct or not—this is real learning.

In conversation, every so often, surgeons share that they are proud to have operated on an enormous number of cases in the previous year. It is not unusual to hear them admit that they were unable to spend much time with their family. (Humorously, it is said that they are saving money to pay the family's psychiatrist.)

Then, of course, follows the obligatory logical question: Why not hire another surgeon in order to divide the work, enjoy it more and spend extra time with your family? Usually, they answer that there is not enough work to share with another person! Indeed, it appears to be a matter of personal ambitions and extreme competitiveness. Yes, surgeons need many cases to increase their experience but if that concept is taken to an extreme, as everything in life, it will end up having a negative impact on their professional and personal life. Surgeons must recognize that they are human beings with basic natural requirements. History shows that every time humans violate the basic biological principles of their existence (sleeping, eating, resting, having fun and having love), the results are disastrous.

COMMON SENSE FIRST

In order to apply knowledge and make a good decision, one must be interested in solving a problem. In surgery, furthermore, the answer to a clinical dilemma is frequently very visible and very obvious. That is why surgeons like to keep in mind:

More is missed by not seeing than by not knowing.

It is typical to witness doctors and surgeons making rounds from the corridor, outside of the patient's room, without ever directly seeing the patient, without seeing their face or talking to them, without viewing the operative area and all of the important parts of the body. It is common to hear doctors discuss sophisticated concepts related with the management of the very sick patient resting in a bed near them. During the discussion, residents and fellows are concerned about not being able to answer questions that the attending surgeons will pose. The attendings might be trying to impress their colleagues with how much they know or they might be attempting to win an old debate related with a controversial pathophysiologic concept.[124] Medical students are anxious because they can hardly understand what the "wise guys" are saying. And, the entire discussion might be based on data provided by a sleepy nurse, taking for granted that everything is accurate. Decisions are made. The discussion is over. The group moves on to the next patient. But one extremely important thing was missed—nobody actually examined the patient!

Patients and their parents wait anxiously for their doctor to make rounds. They are waiting for the doctor to examine them, to make eye contact with them, to answer their questions, relieving their worries and concerns. When that does not happen, they get the feeling that doctors are too busy and their minds are preoccupied with other affairs. Because the doctor does not hear what the mother has to say, does not look at the patient's face nor carefully examine him, the most important, simple and obvious pieces of information remain invisible.

Not too long ago, a child underwent a bladder augmentation. This is when a damaged, congenitally inadequate small bladder is made larger to store enough urine affording the patient an acceptable quality of life. The bladder is augmented with tissue from the colon, small bowel or stomach. During the post-operative

124 Functional changes associated with or resulting from disease or injury.

days and weeks that follow, the bladder is maintained empty with a catheter to protect the suture lines for adequate healing.

On the first post-operative day, the nurse reported that the child was not producing urine through the catheter. Over the phone, the on-call resident assumed that the patient was dehydrated and instructed the nurse to increase the rate of the intravenous fluid. Two hours later, the nurse called the resident again and reported that there was still no urine in the collector bag. The junior resident decided to call the senior resident and he instructed to give the patient a bolus[125] of intravenous fluid. Two boluses later, the patient was again reported as not producing urine. The decision was made to continue administering intravenous fluids and insert a central venous catheter to measure the central venous-pressure, making sure that the patient was not being overloaded with fluids. After the central catheter was inserted, a potent diuretic was administered to increase the flow of urine. The patient became agitated so the attending surgeon was called. Twelve hours after the initial report he finally came to examine the patient and found a very distended abdomen. The attending decided to irrigate the catheter tube and discovered that it was blocked with a mucous plug. After removing the plug, they were able to retain 500 milliliters of urine from the child!

Although the resident obviously possessed knowledge related

125 Large dose of a substance given by injection.

to the management of dehydration and hypovolemia,[126] the event was a simple mechanical error that could have easily been solved using common sense and seeing the patient during the first call. This is the kind of problem that frequently happens in the practice of surgery.

Common sense is not very common.

All physicians have been to a lecture on a sophisticated subject, presented by a supposedly knowledgeable person. The lecturer uses elegant, technical terminology, with multiple abbreviations and crowded tables full of numbers and statistical analysis. Everyone knows that the subject is important and fashionable and they assume that the lecturer is very talented. At the conclusion, everybody agrees that the presentation was "very interesting" but if asked to explain the essence of the lecture, it is unusual to find someone who is able to summarize and simplify it. It is a wonder then how many members of the audience really understood what was presented. Nobody was brave enough (or were they too embarrassed?) to raise a hand and admit to not understanding the lecture in front of an audience that seemed to understand everything.

I read a magazine article referring to the popular movie character Forrest Gump that analyzed how a borderline mentally retarded individual captivated millions and provoked so many positive

126 Diminished volume of circulating blood in the body.

feelings. Part of the answer, the author speculated, was that while Forrest Gump was not exactly intelligent, he had common sense. In comparison, the author suggested, some of the worst atrocities and massive killings in human history (from the Inquisition and the World Wars, to the Holocaust and Vietnam War) were planned and orchestrated by extremely intelligent human beings, against a general common sense. Common sense is like a fresh, simplistic, non-prejudiced analysis of a problem that was otherwise considered complicated.

Simplicity is the ultimate sophistication.

—Leonardo da Vinci

While trying to help young doctors devise a paper, I usually start by inquiring why they want to present the paper. I also challenge them to relay what the central message of their paper is in just two minutes. I demand plain, simple answers, avoiding sophisticated, pseudo-elegant, technical jargon.

Their answer to my first question ("Why do you want to present this paper?") must be sincere. Through the years, I have learned to detect students' sincerity and authenticity. The natural and sincere motivation to write a paper begins in front of a sick patient afflicted with a condition for which there is no good treatment. The next step is a kind of obsessive internal query and search for a solution, followed by the conception of hypotheses that generate a clinical or laboratory research project. When the project is implemented, a young doctor may find a hypothesis to be correct. That is an exhilarating feeling—he is sincerely compelled to tell his colleagues everything about the findings. This is an authentic motivation to write an article.

I firmly believe that without these ingredients, publications and presentations are a waste of time. Unfortunately, many publications and presentations authored by young surgeons were motivated by the desire to achieve other goals, such as being admitted into a training program or being academically promoted. I feel that it is relatively easy to perceive the passion and sincerity of an authentic motivation as opposed to a spurious one, even if the message comes packaged in a very elegant and sophisticated manner.

I consider the answer to my second question ("What is the central message of your presentation?") to be crucial. Sometimes, surprisingly, a young surgeon has trouble answering this succinctly and clearly. It is important to be able to formulate the central theme of a presentation or publication. The theme can be conceived easier if the necessary concepts are kept in mind. (Remember, all the members of the audience should be able to repeat the theme.) Once the central message is clear, it is imperative to try to delete all the material that is irrelevant to the message. Finally, during the presentation, pay close attention to the audience, making a special effort to adapt it to their interest and its possible future practical application.

Reading an interview of Dr. Thomas Starzl (world famous pioneer of liver transplants) on the occasion of receiving the William Ladd Medal, (Ref. 17) I was happily surprised to learn that he declares himself an advocate of clarity and simplicity in writing papers. He even said that he had many problems with editors for his use of a plain, non-sophisticated language. I feel proud to be in the company of such a great surgeon.

EVIDENCE-BASED SURGERY

Occupying a great volume of the current medical and surgical literature are the very popular concepts "evidence-based medicine" and "evidence-based surgery." These terms basically refer to the idea of doctors applying only those operations, maneuvers and treatments known for sure, to be beneficial for a patient. In other words, there must be proof and data to support the claims of certain procedures.

Is "evidence-based medicine and surgery" a new concept? Categorically, no; nevertheless, it is frequently presented like a revelation or something novel. Just what were the great leaders and pioneers of medicine and surgery trying to do in the past? What would they say if they read the current medical literature? The history of medicine and surgery is full of stories of talented, dedicated doctors struggling to do what they thought was good for their patients. They were desperately looking for evidence that those procedures were beneficial. Have doctors been practicing "evidence-based medicine and surgery" throughout the centuries? The answer is mostly, no. However, within their limitations, all doctors have been *trying* to practice evidence-based surgery. But only trying. Then, is "evidence-based medicine and surgery" practiced today? Because it is not easy to obtain such evidence, the answer is, mostly no.

Mathematicians and physicists have been trying for centuries to create carefully worked-out models of biological phenomena and the result is usually a great deal of frustration—research is much easier when the number of variables is limited. In medicine and surgery, for instance, the number of variables is infinite. In the operating room or intensive care unit, the number of variables becomes immeasurable. Even in the most scientifically and technologically advanced environment, in the best institutions in the world, there are infinite numbers of variables. Every patient is different. An operation repeated a thousand times by the same surgeon, includes countless technical maneuvers dealing with specific changing circumstances in the operative field. Human bodies are not machines. Surgeons are not mechanics who can remove a part of the human motor and replace it with a new one, without introducing innumerable factors in each case.

One of the most complicating aspects of "evidence-based surgery" is the inconvenient but true fact that each surgeon performs the same operation in a unique way, with varying degrees of quality. When long-term outcome studies are presented in meetings, the authors attempt to analyze the aspects that determined the final result of the operation. The quality of the surgical technique is never mentioned because it is assumed that it is the same, regardless of the institution and surgeon conducting the operations; yet, surgeons know that operations are performed with multiple degrees of dexterity and expertise. All studies designed to determine the effect of a specific therapeutic modality include numerous subjective steps: evaluating pain, suffering and quality of life represent a serious challenge. All studies are conducted, analyzed and interpreted by human beings, evaluating other human beings, which poses a tendency to be subjective and biased.

Although doctors, by definition, are concerned with the potential benefit or harm inflicted upon patients, the patients and their parents are the ones most concerned with the outcome. Unfortunately, doctors and their patients did not initiate the main motivation of "evidence-based medicine and surgery." Insurance companies, HMOs and government organizations have pushed the concept. These entities are concerned with avoiding complications but it is also true that they are interested in limiting spending in unnecessary treatments. Therefore, the entire system becomes suspicious when the motivation is to save money. It might make sense to reduce spending in some areas but it is rather disheartening to accept.

From a philosophical point of view, the entire concept of

"evidence-based medicine and surgery" becomes much more complicated if, as a parameter, quality of life is introduced. Success in surgery and medicine is accepted when the wound heals well, when the anatomy has been restored, when function returns and symptoms have disappeared. All of these may happen, though, without necessarily improving the patient's quality of life. Examples are everywhere. A complex operation to remove a malignant tumor, followed by chemotherapy and radiotherapy, may be considered successful when a patient's life is prolonged for five years. However, during those years, that individual's quality of life is rarely taken into consideration. By the time the patient is able to evaluate their life throughout those years and give an opinion, it is too late; they have already reached the end. Something similar happens when a tiny mini-premature baby is subjected to sophisticated operations that are deemed successful. As a consequence, the baby may live many years with multiple sequelae, including learning disabilities or cerebral palsy.[127] This makes the whole subject much more intricate and complicated to clarify.

No one has the answer to the multiple challenges that the practice of modern medicine and surgery is presenting. Based on these considerations, doctors are far from reaching the point of being absolutely 100 percent sure that what they do is best for their patients. For many years, there will be an element of personal

127 Disorder usually caused by brain damage occurring at or before birth and marked by muscular impairment.

judgment concerning what is beneficial for patients and that sets up something extremely important: Patients come to doctors, not only for their expertise and dexterity, but also for a human and philosophical perspective—they trust their judgment. This means that being technically good is not good enough. Patients need help from respectable, compassionate, educated, open-minded humanists, capable of understanding human nature and its many manifestations, individuals willing to put the best of their intellect to work.

I believe all doctors are in favor of practicing "evidence-based medicine and surgery"; however, they cannot avoid feeling repulsed by the notion that it is considered a new concept, since it is exactly what every good doctor has been trying to do throughout history. Additionally, doctors are unhappy about the motivations that promoted the concept. "Evidence-based surgery" studies may evaluate long-term results of a specific operation and compare the results of two operations designed to repair the same defect; yet, those studies do not evaluate the literally hundreds of factors of a surgical act, including a surgeon's performance. An operation may be very good when performed by a specific surgeon and extremely poor when conducted by a careless surgeon.

Surgeons may learn and memorize the answers for the examination boards, concerning what is the best course of action in certain situations, but those are relative concepts. For years to come, doctors will practice, attempting to follow scientific principles to the best of their abilities, but their intra-operative decisions will still be based on particular changing circumstances, using subjective, viable and valuable human attributes.

MORTALITY AND MORBIDITY MEETINGS

Most academic hospitals have at least one hour dedicated every week to the retrospective analysis of complications and potential complications that occurred during that week. These gatherings are called "mortality and morbidity meetings" (M&M meetings). The basic philosophy of these events is to encourage surgeons to cultivate a healthy habit (and routine exercise) of asking themselves after each complication, "If I have to do this operation again, how can I prevent another mishap?" In theory, this discussion should not be a defensive discourse. It is not valid for the surgeon to say that they did everything correctly and blame mishaps on patient factors. Instead, surgeons should give the patient the benefit of the doubt, even if there was no misconduct or errors in management.

There are reasons to believe that not all complications during the week are included in the M&M meetings. In fact, some of the most important events, the nearly missed or dangerous episodes occurring in the operating room, are not presented in the meetings. During a surgeon's life in the operating room, there are innumerable times in which a catastrophe nearly takes place. A potential catastrophe is often a consequence of an error; however, for fortunate reasons it was avoided, the patient recovered uneventfully and the case was never discussed in an M&M meeting. (Hopefully, though, it is seared in the surgeon's mind!) The discussions and analysis of possible causes of a complication are centered into sophisticated mechanisms of pathophysiology; yet, sometimes the explanation is found in simple technical errors. Basic, elemental technical errors are not even mentioned because it is assumed that well trained, intelligent, sophisticated professionals (in theory) should avoid those kinds of mistakes.

The only surgeons that do not have complications are those that do not practice surgery.

Consequently, it is extremely desirable and convenient to create a second, more private M&M meeting. This kind of meeting can be conducted, and frequently occurs, between partners of a subspecialty, colleagues with a similar philosophy about the treatment of different conditions, and close friends. For that, it is necessary to develop a degree of confidence and intimacy between colleagues, allowing one to be extremely critical about the other, without producing malicious feelings. When that wonderful friendship and collegiality transpires, it is extremely enjoyable; one goes to the partner knowing that their criticism is unique, valid, sincere and beneficial. It is highly recommended to have this private type of M&M meeting.

Surgeons have the capacity to cure and dramatically change the patient's life—a few millimeters away from the knife is a delicate structure that can be impaired with catastrophic repercussions. Surgeons must learn to live with this duality as part of their every day routine. The practice of good quality surgery requires a high degree of auto-criticism. If the auto-criticism is excessive, the surgeon may suffer so much that his practice becomes a nightmare. But a surgeon without honest auto-criticism may become a "butcher with a license". The key is to find the right balance, as in most human affairs. A young surgeon must make serious efforts to learn about his temperament and recognize if he has the necessary characteristics for this kind of profession.

Then, there is another mortality and morbidity event that occurs in the surgeon's bed at night with the pillow when they cannot sleep, mulling about what could have gone wrong...

God made surgeons with poor memory.

It is only with bad memory that a surgeon can live a happy life, go to work every day with an optimistic attitude, smiling and inspiring confidence in patients, considering the mistakes that were made in the past. It is only with a poor memory that a surgeon can go to work after the loss of a little patient, even when the loss was beyond their control. Surgeons must continuously analyze their performance retrospectively, thinking of better ways to work, without any of the paralyzing anxiety.

*****

Medical and surgical literature is full of triumphant and successful reports. It is not unexpected to read a paper describing a "new procedure" or a "new treatment" because old ones "were not good." One often wonders why there is talk about a "new procedure" when all of the papers from the "old" operations reported excellent results. Suspiciously, most papers talk about success even though new operations and new therapeutic methodologies are always being sought. Where are the reports of the failures? Where are the reports of the complications? If a doctor writes a paper about his newly designed operation, then he is morally obligated to disclose every detail of the operation. Even if everyone assumes the new operation was highly successful, the doctor must inform colleagues about the problems that his patients endured.

During my training at Children's Hospital Boston, I learned from Dr. Kenneth Welch, a procedure to repair a condition called pectus excavatum.[128] The operation basically consisted of performing

128 Deformity consisting of a depressed chest wall.

a sub-perichondrial resection[129] of the costal cartilages[130] related to the deformity of the sternum.[131] By doing that, the sternum becomes a very mobile structure. The sternum was then surgically fractured and fixed in a desired position, correcting the deformity.

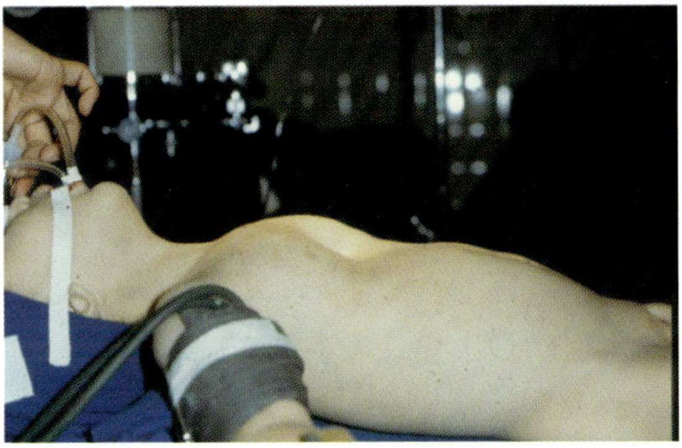

(Fig. 4) Pectus excavatum; A chest wall deformity

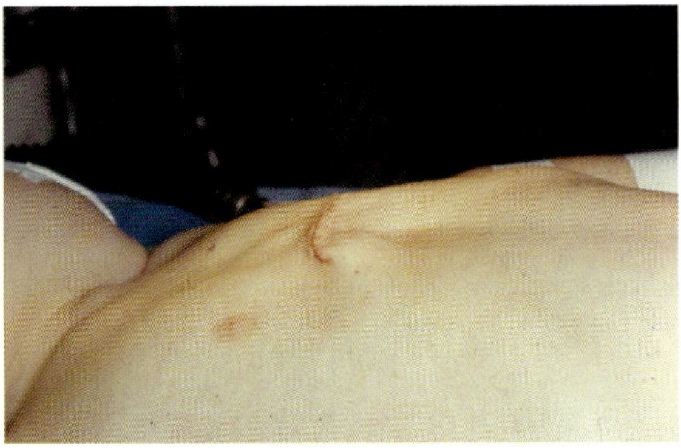

(Fig. 5) A repaired pectus excavatum; Immediate post-operative results were spectacularly good

The immediate results from this operation were spectacularly positive. I also learned that the operation was easier to perform on

129 Surgical removal of the fibrous membrane covering the surface of cartilage.

130 The cartilage forming the anterior continuation of a rib.

131 A long flat bone, articulating with the cartilages of the first seven ribs and with the clavicle, forming the middle part of the anterior wall of the thorax. Breastbone.

younger patients. I went back to Mexico and found that pediatric surgeons were not familiar with this operation—there was only one publication in the Mexican medical literature related to the treatment of this condition in adolescents and young adults.

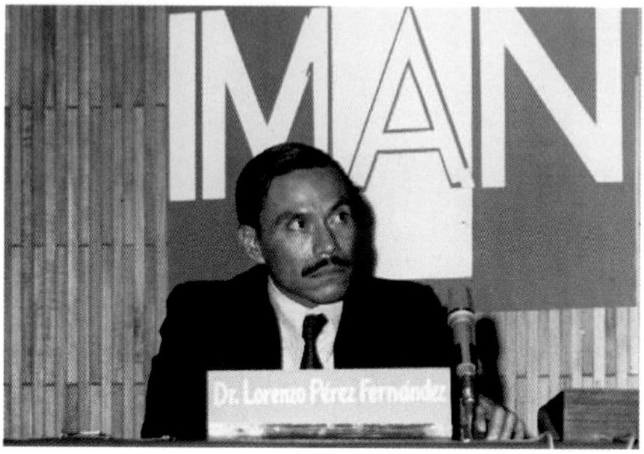

Dr. Lorenzo Perez-Fernandez, an excellent friend

At IMAN, Dr. Lorenzo Perez-Fernandez (my friend and fellow surgeon) and I took over the responsibility of operating on all the patients with pectus excavatum. As we started doing that procedure, more patients with the same condition came to our hospital. Being young and ambitious, it was very flattering to receive invitations to lecture on the subject and operate on many patients. We published our early experience and were very proud of our results.

Fortunately, because Dr. Perez-Fernandez and I were in Mexico we were able to stay in contact with most of our patients for several years. It was with complete horror that we saw many of our "successes" suffer from a lack of growth of the entire chest, not only in the area of the cartilage resection. (Fig. 6) The deformity and lack of growth was far worse in the younger patients! I searched

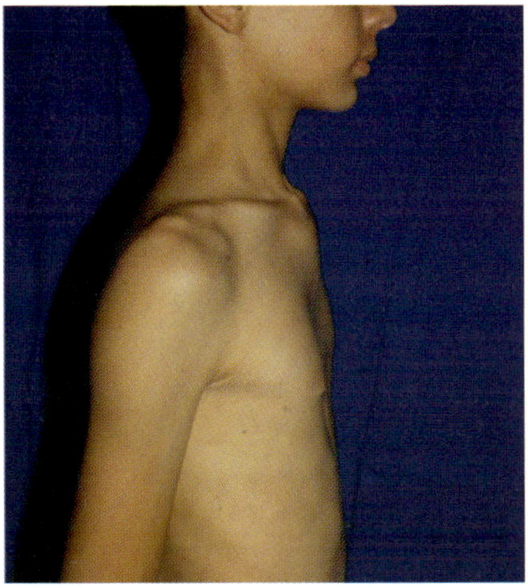

(Fig. 6) Long term follow up showed a remarkable lack of growth of the chest

and searched but could not find a publication indicating that this happened anywhere else. I initiated a research project to investigate if the resection of the costal cartilages provoked the deformity. For that, I invited five enthusiastic, last year medical students of the Military Medical School to join me. The work would be their mandatory graduation thesis.

Because laboratory research in Mexico was extremely complicated due to the lack of resources in those years, the students and I liked to say that the "ethical committee" (formed by all of us) approved the project and that the financial support came from a grant obtained from the "Peña Foundation." With our combined resources, each one of the students bought two puppies of the same litter. The plan was to remove the costal cartilages in five puppies while the other five received a similar operation without removing the cartilages. We would observe all puppies growing for six months, evaluating them clinically, taking x-rays every month. The operations were carried out at the Military Medical School.

The school, however, refused to house the animals for that period unless somebody paid for the expenses. So, I encouraged the students to test their girlfriends' devotion and asked them to adopt and care for two puppies each, during the six month study. Our protocol included taking an x-ray of the animals every month to monitor the growth of their chests but the question was where, how and who will pay for so many x-rays? Following an old code I learned in the military, "It is better to apologize than to ask for permission," a decision was made. Every month, at night, the puppies were sneaked into the radiology department of the Central Military Hospital for chest films. After six months, the clinical and radiologic observations confirmed our suspicions. At an early age, the resection of the costal cartilages produced a severe lack of growth and development of the entire chest! The results were so obvious and grotesque that it did not require statistical analysis.

Our experience was presented at the annual meeting of the American Academy of Pediatrics) in San Francisco. I was amazed to hear that surgeons with more experience on the subject say they never encountered that complication. Our paper was not accepted for publication because of the "limited number of animals" in our research. Years later, working in New York, I decided to persist

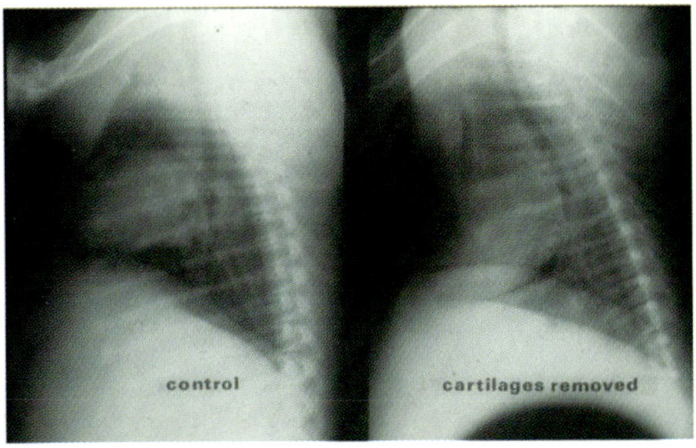

(Fig.7) Lateral films of the animal's chest comparing those with intact cartilages (left) with those with cartilages removed (right)

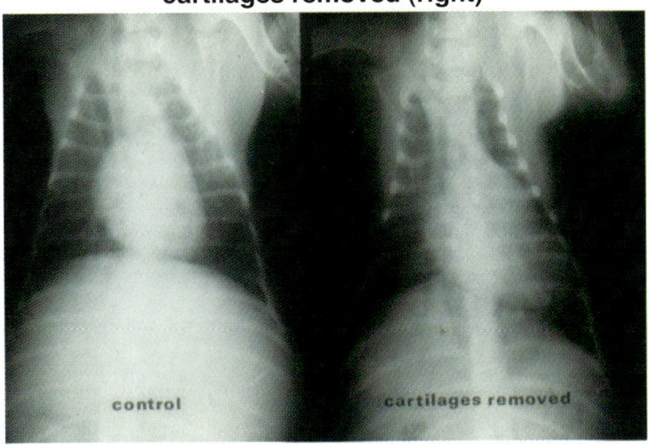

(Fig.8) Same animals in anterior-posterior views

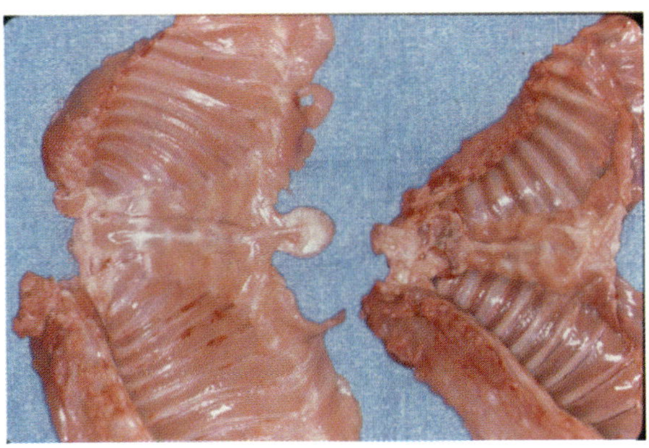

(Fig. 9) The cartilage resection affected the growth of the entire chest as shown here; Left: specimen in a control animal; Right: animal that underwent cartilage resection

and repeat the study, using 40 rabbits. The results were just as spectacular as those observed in dogs. Finally, our paper was accepted for publication in *Pediatric Surgery International* (Ref. 18) but received very few comments. After that, Dr. Donald Nuss (from Norfolk, Virginia) designed a new, less invasive procedure without a cartilage resection. (Ref. 19)

Many years after all of this, some senior surgeons (and former advocates of the cartilage resection) approached me, "Alberto, you were right, we have seen patients with that kind of late sequelae." In fact, currently, there is some litigation related with similar problems.

It is not so bad to make mistakes; the problem is not recognizing them.

A COMPREHENSIVE REVIEW

In these modern times, surgeons attend big meetings to learn more about their profession and the sophisticated advances in surgery: transplantation, fetal surgery, basic science research subjects and robotics. When the meeting is over, it is not unusual for a surgeon to feel a bit overwhelmed, realizing that science and technology is progressing extremely fast. So fast, that it appears there is no way to keep up with it. Day-by-day, surgeons sense that they are lagging behind, becoming more deficient and ignorant about so many of the new emerging developments. It is hard to keep up with it all!

A good way to decrease a little bit of this anxiety is for a surgeon to select one particular topic in surgery, based purely on the desire to satisfy a very sincere personal curiosity. (It could even be considered a hobby used to "recharge you batteries.") The idea is to select a topic, not with the specific purpose of winning the

Nobel Prize, not with the expectation to be invited to give lectures all over the world, not to be promoted academically, but simply because of the intrinsic pleasure obtained from learning about a condition and the evolution of various ways to treat that condition. Gradually, without noticing, the surgeon becomes a real expert on the subject.

That kind of review requires a deep exhaustive and comprehensive reading and analysis of the available literature. Try to read all of the literature ever written on that particular topic. It is a fascinating experience. I said *try* to read all of the literature because it is virtually impossible to do so. For serendipitously mysterious reasons life took me on unexpected paths and I have become an "expert" in pediatric colorectal surgery. After many years of practice and reading, I still cannot claim that I have read all of the papers ever written on the subject, even though I keep trying.

The comprehensive bibliography review must be carried out slowly (without being in a hurry), savoring every single paper. The reward is in the process, not in the result. In the process one may discover fascinating facts: A surgeon might appreciate the contrast between himself and a surgeon practicing 300 years ago. Anxieties of the surgeons of the old times might be revealed. Another surgeon might admire the way papers were written in the 1800s, full of personal anecdotes, versus the way they are written now. A review might include, perhaps, several thousand papers related to a subject giving the surgeon insight and some moral authority.

One may even be surprised to find that only very few are important enough to be distinguished as seminal, relevant original papers, that have actually influenced the knowledge and treatment of a particular condition. A comprehensive review also uncovers a tendency humans have to repeat what others have already said. Very few things are new.

One can also learn how the so-called "advances in surgery" move in a pendulum-like fashion. From a wide perspective, humans appear to be very predictable. One specific "advance" becomes popular at some time, is abandoned and eventually resuscitated and presented again as new. This teaches surgeons to be enthusiastic but cautious when evaluating a "new" development in surgery. Many times surgeons thought they were writing about a new concept only to find that it was actually a repetition of something that somebody said 100 years before!

A paper written by a bold pioneer daring to challenge conventional wisdom for the first time is suddenly exposed. He may be right or wrong but he is the first person to express doubt. If correct, he becomes one of the few that will be remembered. The exhaustive literary review may show how pathophysiologic, anatomic and embryologic concepts accepted by generations of physicians, are still present, untouched and rarely questioned. Even in this 21st century, surgical books remain full of "sacred" concepts written many years ago by a famous, self-confident surgeon. Those concepts are still there simply because nobody has challenged *their* veracity.

Those that wrote papers without an important fundamental message in mind (unfortunately too many to count) can also be detected with a comprehensive review. Most likely, their papers were written with spurious motivations. It is relatively easy to distinguish authors that wrote about something they really knew and dealt with every day from those that wrote something based mainly in theory. Very few surgeons have the time to perform this kind of deep study. When a surgeon becomes an "important professor" it is precisely then that he has less time to do this. It is most probable for a surgeon to be able to do that when he is not so famous and not so busy.

There are papers that have been quoted in the medical literature thousands of times—everybody mentions them but very few have actually read the originals. Most pediatric surgeons know, for instance, that Cameron Haight operated on the first patient with esophageal atresia through an extrapleural approach,[132] successfully performing an end-to-end esophageal anastomosis. (Ref. 20) But very few have read his original paper. I highly recommended reading that paper to learn how in 1939, Cameron Haight performed an anastomosis of the esophagus in a newborn baby without intravenous fluids, without endotracheal intubation, without respirators and without antibiotics....

132 Situated outside the area of the chest that includes the lining of the chest cavity.

MORAL AUTHORITY

Surgeons are divided into those who talk about surgery and those who operate.

Moral authority is a form of power that is not based in specific documents, contracts, degrees, titles and academic ranks, number of publications, money or political activity. It is a power that peers and colleagues recognize in a person based on performance. It is granted and acknowledged in spontaneous, non-mandatory ways. In the military, moral authority is obtained by being the first to fight, the best fighter, the bravest, most protective and helpful leader. I believe that surgeons recognize the moral authority of another colleague by watching him in the operating room, making rounds, seeing patients in the clinic and teaching residents. The rest is theory. Moral authority is the fundamental ingredient of a good chief of surgery.

Surgeons attend many surgical meetings and hear wonderful

lectures. Some of the lectures are so good that they spark a certain degree of skepticism about their authenticity. The only way to know the answer to that question is to visit the lecturer and observe him in his own environment for several days. Being there with him, it is possible to learn that, in actuality, the man is even more admirable than initially thought. Unfortunately, the exact opposite is possible as well: *everything* presented in the lecture was completely theoretical.

In some countries, when surgeons are appointed chief of surgery, they think they have gained certain privileges. One such privilege consists in not going to the clinic to see patients. Another may be to only operate on certain types of cases or not to operate at all! This, I think, is the "beginning of the end" in terms of their moral authority. If a chief does not feel like operating any longer, decides not to see patients and not to follow his patients, he should move laterally. He should stop being an active chief just to receive some sort of honorary title and recognition and try not to interfere with the activities of those still on the battlefield. It is astounding to see some chiefs operate on patients but never examine them in the clinic; instead, young attending surgeons tend to the patients in the clinic and another group of younger surgeons write the papers (always with the obligation to write the chief's name as an author!). In some socialized medicine type of environments, where there is no material incentive for seeing patients, most doctors consider the clinic outpatient department to be like a punishment.

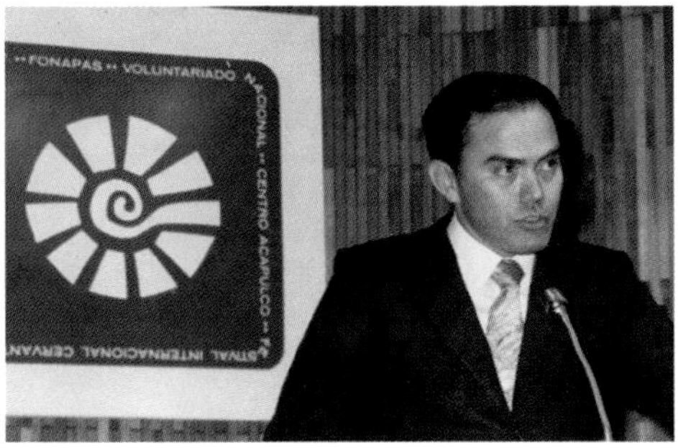

Dr. Peña as Director of National Institute of Pediatrics, Mexico

At some point in my life, while in Mexico, I was offered the job of director of INP. The offer was too flattering for my ego and I accepted. I fantasized that I could administrate the hospital, continue being academically productive and operate. A year and a half later I resigned the position and went back to my job as a chief of surgery. Three important episodes contributed to my resignation.

One afternoon when I was in my huge office, concentrating on the multiple problems that came through my desk, my secretary notified me that a first year surgical resident wanted to talk to me. The young resident, Antonio Gallardo, came into my office claiming to be the messenger of the chief surgical resident and all the other surgical residents, extending the most cordial invitation to make rounds with them. Then it hit me—I had not been making rounds with them for at least two months. Feeling embarrassed, I left everything and walked with the resident toward the surgical floor. On our way, the resident spoke to me with a little bit of hesitation, "Dr. Peña, the reason why I applied to this pediatric surgical training program is because of your reputation as a surgeon. I wanted to learn from you. I have been here for about six months now and I have not seen you operate once." Silence. The message was very clear. I was not able to sleep well that night.

The second incident unfolded one day at noon while the kitchen workers were threatening to go on strike if their demands were not fulfilled. They were refusing to serve lunch to 700 hospital workers. There I was, with less than optimal knowledge of syndicalism, worker's rights and labor laws, trying to convince them to be reasonable and serve lunch so we could continue our dialogue afterwards. In the middle of the heated discussion I got a call from the operating room that my patient was under anesthesia waiting for me. I said a few last words to the workers and walked upstairs to the operating room. When I entered the OR I saw the intubated child and could not remember what operation I was supposed to do. I had to reference the medical record and find my notes. Thankfully, the operation went well but again the message was very clear. More insomnia that night....

During one of my visits with Dr. Judah Folkman in Boston, the third episode took place. It was always refreshing to have a conversation with Dr. Folkman. We were discussing people that deserve and receive veneration. So, I asked him to name a person, dead or alive, that he admired most. I was nearly floored by his reply, "I admire Tiger Woods."

His answer surprised me, not because Tiger Woods may not

deserve admiration but because, as far as I knew, Dr. Folkman was not interested in sports. I urged Dr. Folkman to explain why he admired Tiger Woods so much. "Because he is able to focus on what he is doing."

Dr. Folkman proceeded to tell me that for several years he toiled as surgeon-in-chief while simultaneously running a growing, impressive research laboratory. He, therefore, decided to resign as surgeon-in-chief and work full time in the lab. Something, he admitted, that should have happened years earlier. Meditating on this, when I returned to Mexico, I resigned as director of INP and promised myself never to accept that kind of job in the future.

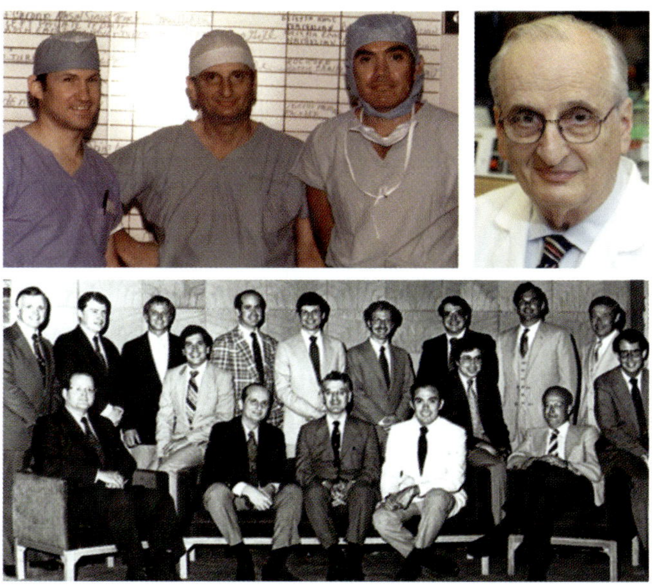

Above left: Robert Shamberger, Judah Folkman, and Alberto Peña, Boston; Above right: Dr. Judah Folkman; Below: Back row from left to right: Willis Williams, Ted Ballantine, Tim Canty, C.D. Smith, Jay Vacanti, Gerald Weinberg, Richard Harmel, David Tapper, Arnold Coran; Front row from left to right: John Noseworthy, Pedro Rosello, Judah Folkman, Howard Snyder, Alberto Peña, Arvin Phillipart, Marshall Schwartz

THE MAGIC OF CREATIVITY AND THE POWER OF AN IDEA

One of the most sophisticated intellectual activities of the human brain is creativity. It is mysterious because it happens in a quite spontaneous, unintentional way and not necessarily because one tries to be creative. Simply, creativity happens or it does not.

A happy oyster does not produce a pearl.

—Rubem Alves

Under demanding, stressful circumstances, anybody might be creative. Creativity may actually be a kind of survival tool and, in fact, it has been so throughout man's history. Sometimes it takes pain, suffering and desperation to generate a creative solution for a problem. That kind of creativity is a fascinating subject; however, for the purpose of this book, mainly related with the subject of surgery, I will discuss another type of creativity not induced by stressfully desperate circumstances.

*****

Everybody can be creative but there are some individuals who create things that truly influence the lives of most human beings. They are revered as great geniuses, individuals who contributed to the progress of humankind and changed the course of history. It is intriguing to find that these extraordinary beings shared a sort of unexplainable, burning curiosity that was more powerful than anything else in their lives. These individuals were obsessed with trying to meet the challenge of a specific dilemma. The answer did not necessarily bring them money, power or titles. Many times, it brought nothing but difficulties, but still they could not resist the temptation to not think about that one specific question. This is what I call an authentic motivation to investigate. A person can investigate something mentally or with scientific instruments, following a specific methodology or not at all.

When Charles Darwin accepted the position as a biologist on the HMS Beagle, a boat that the British government sent to inspect the coast of South America, he was hired to do a sort of census of the potential natural resources they found. Darwin had his own agenda in mind. During his years on that ship, he was provoked by a burning curiosity to find patterns and explanations as to why many species of plants and animals shared similarities and dissimilarities. He returned to England with thousands of specimens. If somebody had looked at his baggage of specimens, they would have thought that he was the most impractical and crazy person in the world. Most people, though, did not care about what he was collecting and observing.

Darwin spent many years examining his collection trying to come up with a theory to explain such diversity. He did not publish a single essay about his ideas during all those years. In fact, he was afraid that his ideas would provoke serious turmoil in society (as it turned out). He was not interested in an academic title or money; he happened to belong to a family with enough resources to live well anyway. It was his all-consuming curiosity that kept him busy, doing all that research in his own home on his own time. Similar stories about Einstein, Newton, Galileo and many others could be discussed.

Everyday, surgeons examine patients with problems from operations and complications that, many times, cannot be cured. This is a source of an enormous number of legitimate questions and potential research projects. But if the surgeon does not feel a sincere urge to ponder these questions because it would otherwise become an obsession and if he is not fascinated by the analysis of the question, it would be a waste of time. I do not think he would be able to do significant research and make valuable contributions to science and technology.

I have had many conversations with young surgeons who have an impressive curriculum—very young doctors with 10, 12 or 15 basic science research papers published, all of them with sophisticated titles not easy for me to understand. I asked why they investigated a particular subject and the answer, time and again, has been, "Because I was recommended to do research so that I could be accepted in the training program." It appears as if they did not possess an authentic motivation to conduct research. Again, I believe that this is a waste of time and resources.

There are a few pediatric surgeons who are authentically motivated to investigate at a basic scientific level. One of them was Dr. Judah Folkman. He actually "suffered" being chief of surgery for about ten years before he finally decided to work full time in his laboratory. He was an excellent chief of surgery but a question still remains: If he had resigned ten years earlier to completely dedicate himself to research, could he have been more productive and perhaps won the first Nobel Prize given to a pediatric surgeon?

Creativity does not necessarily result in winning a Nobel Prize or advancements that affect the entire world. Creativity may end up in small but important contributions in the practice. Most of the surgeons that I know have new ideas, ideas that emerge unexpectedly and very easily. The problem they face is in the implementation of these ideas. From mind to laboratory to clinic, ideas have to be proven. It is the logistical aspect that represents a major obstacle. It may be necessary to study hundreds of patients and implement the necessary statistical analysis of the results, which takes time and dedication. Because of the money involved, the time required and specific circumstances in the life of an already overexerted surgeon, many ideas never crystallize into real research projects.

Many young, academic pediatric surgeons search for a job with a guarantee of being able to devote 50% of their time to research. There are some surgeons who have actually spent half of their time in the laboratory and half their time in clinical practice but I still have serious reservations about what that concept means. A busy clinical surgeon, fully dedicated to clinical surgery, spends 35-40 years of his life repeatedly operating on the same conditions, attempting to improve surgical techniques to avoid complications and obtain better results. At the end of those years, being honest with himself, the clinical surgeon realizes that he never really mastered *all* surgical procedures. This is particularly true if he is trying to be a master surgeon in multiple areas. No one can ever really claim to reach perfection in the art of surgery.

If, in addition, operative time is reduced by 50% it is fair to assume that it would provoke a double anxiety unless standards of quality are compromised. A possible solution for a surgeon wanting to practice clinical surgery 50% of the time is to take on a very narrow, specific subspecialty. It is not easy to operate with good standards of quality in all areas of general pediatric surgery while dedicating only 50% of the time to surgery. Surgery does not permit that. Surgery is unforgiving; it demands full attention and dedication.

There are literally thousands of basic scientists who have dedicated their lives to one specific subject, pulling the string, going deeper and deeper, finding more and more fascinating, unanswered questions and becoming more and more intrigued the deeper they research. It seems that one entire lifetime is not enough for them and they eventually retire or die with the feeling that they left a job undone. If that were true, having dedicated their entire life to study, imagine how it would be if they were limited to research only 50% of their time. Believing that they can dedicate half of their time to research and be a productive, creative scientist is disrespectful to the scientific activity. The same follows for surgeons. It is conceivable that very specifically talented young surgeons could develop a line of research intimately related to the specific type of operation they perform but they cannot fantasize that they can still do liver resections, esophageal replacements, pull-throughs and cloacae repairs while spending half of their time in research.

Nothing is stronger than an idea whose time has come.

—Victor Hugo

It is equally mysterious and fascinating how an idea is born and the possibility of that idea to impact science, technology and history. Heroes, thinkers, philosophers, scientists and geniuses who have changed history did not have to write a research protocol. They did not have to spend many hours, days and weeks meticulously writing a grant application adhering to the rules and specifications of the institutional review board (IRB)[133] to be granted the approval to proceed with their project. They did not have to ask for permission from an ethical committee or obtain a master's degree in business administration to write the financial budget for their project. Even in modern times, I believe that the power of an idea remains fundamental but its realization requires overcoming several legal, bureaucratic, academic, sometimes political and economic barriers. Due to all of the obstacles imposed on the potential researcher, many ideas never see the light

Ironically, sometimes rather poor ideas have been successfully implemented because they were wrapped in an impeccable protocol adhering to all of the requirements of the modern scientific methodology. These ideas satisfy the bureaucratic requirements and are presented with a meticulously elaborated business plan using an excellent technical jargon. Sometimes, the wrapping is so complicated that it is very tough to know exactly what is the most important part.

There are many individuals in the medical and scientific field who become experts in the scientific method and all of the bureaucratic, academic and financial requirements considered key

133 Organizational committee that reviews and approves biomedical research that uses humans as subjects.

to achieve an approval and grant for a research project. Some of these individuals have very good ideas while others, although intelligent, have no good ideas. Some use their knowledge to criticize or even destroy protocols written by less experienced professionals. There are many doctors and professionals who have great ideas but are unaccustomed with the necessary methodology to overcome the barriers of implementing their ideas. They could learn the methodology but it tends to be complex and time consuming for an otherwise busy and overwhelmed doctor.

In an ideal world, a proposal could be presented in a couple of pages with very simple words and concise definitions of goals. Individuals familiar with the subject could determine whether the idea is worthwhile. If the proposal is considered sound, they could encourage the author to proceed through the rather painful process of working in the budget, IRB, ethical concerns, using the adequate jargon, a statistic methodology, academic requirements, literature review and author's copyrights. Then, the institutions in charge of promoting and supporting research for the public benefit could facilitate the process for the basic idea to be executed. If the proposal is initially considered to have no potential merit, the author would be discouraged to continue. In that way, doctors, institutions and administrators could save a lot of time and resources by working together more effectively.

Of course, doctors are aware of prevailing reasons why an IRB, an ethical committee, scientific protocol and a financial budget are mandatory. As a matter of fact, it is highly unlikely that those procedures will ever be simplified and easier to understand and perform in the future. Certainly, it is discouraging to have a conversation with a colleague about what seems to be a fascinating and beautiful idea and, rather than discussing and encouraging the idea, the colleague inquires, "How do you expect to handle the IRB? Where are you going to get the money?"

This is a plea for those familiar with the scientific method and the bureaucratic strategy to apply their knowledge to assist those who have good ideas but are unfamiliar with the process. This is a plea for such individuals to encourage such ideas, rather than interfere with them. This is a plea to many doctors who have valuable ideas to not feel so intimidated by all of the barriers and proceed with their intentions.

In many of the medical institutions of the world there is a position called Chief of Investigation or Chief of Research. Frequently, very distinguished researchers with an impeccable background and curriculum vitae occupy those jobs. Sometimes, however, experts of the bureaucratic process and protocol hold these positions. The Chief of Research could be an individual who has very few ideas and uses the position as a source of power, sanctioning a specific, rather humble protocol in an implacable way simply because the person presenting the protocol did not follow the methodological rules. When this occurs, many young individuals become discouraged.

The Chief of Research of any institution should be considered and defined as a post to promote investigation and stimulate young people to improve the outcome of treatments. In order to begin new research projects and creative ideas, the Chief of Research should use all of their knowledge and experience to help others to obtain IRB approval, adequately prepare grant applications and follow the correct methodology.

ETHICAL COMMITTEES

During man's entire history, there have been healers, witches, shamans and doctors (with or without a title) practicing some activity aimed to improve man's quality of life. When life and death dilemmas were at hand, a group was called upon to assess the situation. That group typically included the patient, close relatives, senior members of the community, religious leaders and a doctor. Ultimately, the group came to a decision that was generally accepted by the community. As one can expect, throughout history, the concepts of "good" and "bad" varied greatly depending on various world cultures. What was "good" in one place or time could be "bad" in another place or time.

Ethics is defined as a discipline concerned with what is "good" and "bad" with moral duty and obligation. There may be no other profession besides medicine that poses so many ethical and moral dilemmas. In this profession, physicians implement treatments that can provoke serious damage to patients. Physicians have to make decisions about what is "good" and "bad" for human beings, understanding that it depends very much on ever-changing diverse social circumstances and limitations imposed by the law.

In modern times, lawyers have invaded the territory of morals and medical ethics, more and more. Perhaps this is because it is much easier to adhere to laws rather than making decisions with uncertain moral and ethical consequences. This is particularly true in this era of constant litigation. Increasingly, lawyers tell doctors not to impose personal views on their patients or their parents. They say the patient and the parents should decide, and have the right to decide, about the type of treatment that they receive. But the truth is, even if doctors do not want it, their opinions are and always will be, extremely powerful and influential to a patient. Most patients have come to expect that from their doctors. Doctors present therapeutic alternatives and their consequences in various ways, describing scenarios that weigh consciously or subconsciously upon the patient's decision. Even when showing cold statistics, doctors can use variations in their language to influence the patient in one direction or another. It is practically impossible not to shape the patient's decision. After all, good doctors always ask themselves what they would do if they were the patients or if it was their family. So many times, their patients ask that very question.

*****

One of my patients with a serious congenital anorectal malformation also suffered from an orthopedic defect.[134] The patient's mother wanted me to suggest an orthopedic surgeon whom I trusted and requested a consultation with him, taking advantage of the fact that her child had to stay in the hospital to recuperate from my operation. I was happy to grant the mother's request. Three days later, during my routine daily rounds, I was surprised to find the mother crying. She told me that the surgeon I recommended had examined her son and reported that the child's condition would most likely deteriorate to the point of not being able to walk. The surgeon proceeded to present an operation that could possibly avoid that outcome but said there were no guarantees—it was a major procedure with serious potential for morbidity that included, ironically, not being able to walk. The mother specifically asked the surgeon what he would do in that situation and he answered that he would do whatever she wanted. The mother felt desolated and did not know what to do.

I met with the orthopedic surgeon about the mother and his first reaction was to say that he told her the truth so that she could decide what to do. I expressed to him that I adhered to the concept of advising my patients' parents with what *I* believe to be the best possible treatment and what *I* would do if the patient were my child. The doctor graciously accepted my suggestion and went to

134 Problems occurring in the supporting structures of the body (bones, joints, ligaments, muscles, etc).

share his preference of treatment with the mother. That significantly relieved the mother's anxiety and helped her to make a decision for her child.

*****

It was in my professional time that ethical committees were created in hospitals. Ethical committees are multidisciplinary bodies composed of a broad spectrum of personnel (including physicians, nurses, social workers, priests and others) that address moral and ethical issues within the hospital. I was excited to learn that doctors would have a specific forum to voice all of their concerns, doubts and hesitations about patients. In general, though, I must say that I have been disappointed with every interaction I have had with ethical committees. In most of my encounters, although very professional, the members of the committee did not discuss essential ethical issues but instead maintained what was legally correct! It is upsetting to think that many of the ethical committees were actually created to prevent a hospital from being sued. To avoid such problems, these committees provide legal technical assistance instead of discussing pertinent issues.

It will not be easy for doctors to change the current way medicine is practiced, particularly in this era of the so-called industrialized world. I predict, for the coming decades (and perhaps centuries), the doctor will remain an important fixture in the decision-making process of moral and ethical medical issues in society. Considering that doctors are always involved in making decisions about human welfare, they should be ethicists by definition. Nobody denies the importance of including in the doctor's curriculum, the many hours dedicated to the various ethical and moral issues that will be confronted during their professional life.

In pediatric surgery, the prenatal diagnosis of serious congenital anomalies is already presenting very serious ethical dilemmas. Doctors cannot relinquish the right and obligation to participate in those decisions. In the future, doctors will face much more complex ethical dilemmas. For instance, doctors will reach the point in which they will be able to manipulate genetic material, in turn, posing serious quandaries for society as a whole. Doctors' participation will be extremely important.

Hopefully, doctors can solve the moral problems in their practice before they reach the legal arena. When moral issues are legalized the whole subject becomes rigid, bureaucratized and inflexible, eventually running into the danger of becoming paradoxically unethical.

THE FUTURE

It is easier to be a historian than a prophet.

—overheard from a pathologist

What I have expressed here is in no way a prediction but a wish list. As a human being, I believe that the best philosophical position is an optimistic one. Even when I know that this assumption is based purely on faith, I am still an incurable optimist. I want to reiterate my belief that new generations will bring a fresh, creative and innovative mentality, capable of implementing solutions for the multiple dilemmas affecting human kind. I believe this to be true for all kinds of human activities. What is coming in the near future is the best ever.

I would love to see medical professors dedicate more time to the vocational orientation and selection of individuals with the necessary skills to practice the art of surgery, choosing candidates who possess a good attitude, good temperament, passion and a sincere interest in improving the quality of a human life. I would put less interest in only detecting those individuals with the most intelligence.

I look forward to seeing a better doctor-patient relationship. This, I believe, could come as an upshot of the better selection of doctors. Good doctors establish a humane relationship with patients, hopefully influencing the patient's perception of the care they have received. Amazingly, the fact that a country is extremely developed and economically rich does not necessarily result in the patient's perception that they receive better care; in fact, it seems to be almost the opposite. I hope that medicine and surgery can shift from a litigating, bureaucratic and highly commercialized doctor-patient relationship into a more respectful, affectionate, responsible, faithful one.

Advertising the triumphs and successes of medicine and surgery, with the specific purpose of attracting more patients, increasing the economical rewards and making medicine a business, induces patients to have the wrong expectations about a doctor's capacity to cure. I have the feeling that even when doctors do not specifically lie to the patients, they do not offer the whole truth. When operating on a mini-preemie and trying to keep the baby alive at all costs, surgeons leave the parents the decision about life and death, not telling them the whole story about a possible future for a child with brain damage. Perhaps the paradigm must shift from one that emphasizes the value of life at all costs into another that emphasizes the quality of life. Together, doctors and patients should learn to interpret nature's design from the biological or the religious point of view. Human beings must accept death as part of the life process.

There is a big difference between curing and prolonging the act of dying.

The future will bring extraordinary scientific and technologic advances and with that, humans will face unpredictable and unexpected moral dilemmas. Hopefully, doctors will maintain a high degree of moral authority, credibility and respectfulness to be able to remain a prominent figure in the discussion and solution of future tribulations.

Guided by the same optimistic attitude, my message to the new generations of doctors is to first, be sincere about their vocation. In my own specialty, I recommend that young doctors ask themselves (before making a vocational decision) if they are sure about being deeply interested in performing operations on children. If they feel a passion about it, if they cannot see themselves practicing another specialty, if they consider it an honor and privilege to be a pediatric surgeon, if all of those premises are true, then I suggest they embrace this beautiful profession full on and not pay much attention to pessimistic voices. Do not be intimidated by the increasing litigating atmosphere, do not worry about the financial future, do not use valuable mental energy to study the complicated, intricate bureaucracy that appears to be invading the practice of surgery. The essence of medicine and surgery is to focus mental energy and skills to cure patients, to improve the quality of life of those that cannot be cured and give honest and sincere advice to patients and their parents. I firmly believe that this promotes a better relationship between patients and doctors. The new generation of doctors should not be simple witnesses of the extraordinary evolution that will occur. These new doctors should be active protagonists and play a vital, fundamental role in the intricate ethical dilemmas and the consecutive political decisions to come.

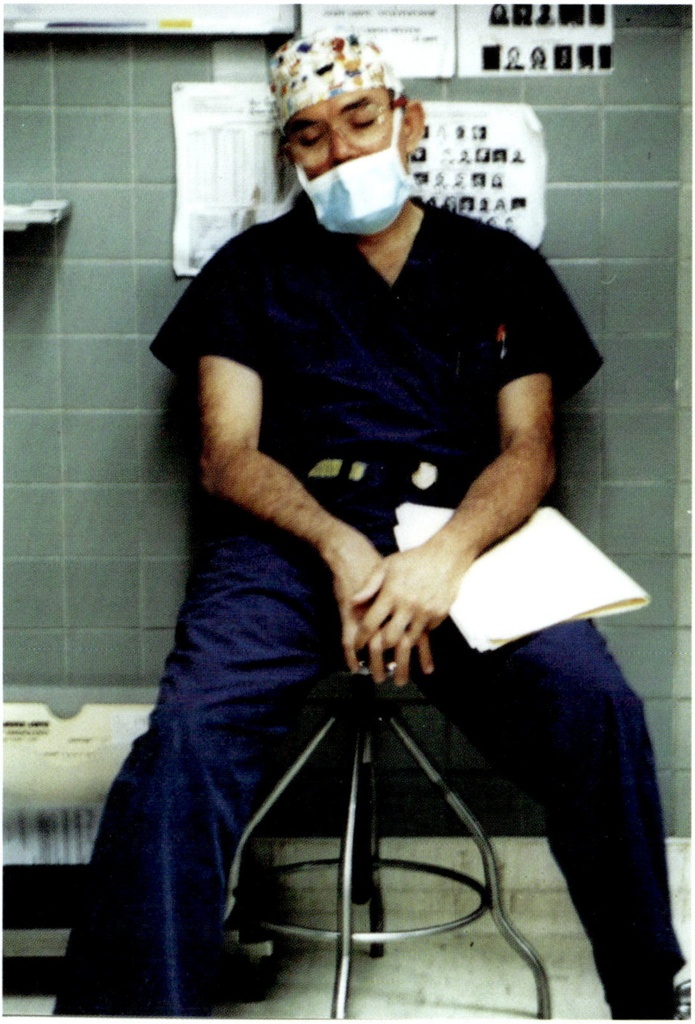

Men have not exhausted the questions,

rather questions exhausted many men.

— Santiago Ramón y Cajal

REFERENCES

1. Gross, Robert E., *The Surgery of Infancy and Childhood*. W. B. Saunders Company. Philadelphia, London 1953

2. Randolph, J.G.: History of the Section of Surgery, the American Academy of Pediatrics the first 25 years (1948-1973). J Ped Surg 34, No 5 Suppl 1 p.p. 3-18, 1999

3. Gross, Robert E., *An Atlas of Children's Surgery*. W.B. Saunders Company. Philadelphia, London, Toronto. 1970

4. Gross, Robert E., Hubbard, John P.: "Surgical Ligation of Patent Ductus Arteriosus: A Report of First Successful Case." J. AMA. 112:729 (1939)

5. Gross, Robert E.: "A Surgical Approach for Ligation of a Patent Ductus Arteriosus". New Engl. J Med 220:510 (1939)

6. Gross, Robert E.: "Surgical Management of the Patent Ductus Arteriosus" Ann Surg., 110:321 (1939)

7. Gibbons Jr., John H.: "Application of a Mechanical Heart and Lung Apparatus to Cardiac Surgery" Minn. Med. 37:171 (1954)

8. Lillehei, C. Walton, Cohen, Morley, Warden, Herbert E., Ziegler, Newell R., Varco, Richard L.: "The Result of Direct Vision Closure of Ventricular Septal Defects in 8 Patients by Means of Controlled Cross Circulation. Surg. Gynec & Obst. 101:447 (1955)

9. Hendren, W.H., Cloaca, The most severe degree of imperforate anus: experience with 195 cases. Ann Surg. 228 (3) 331-346, 1998

10. Björk, V.O., Present Indications for Space-Diminishing Procedures after Pulmonary Resections for Tuberculosis. Acta Chir Scand 112(6):454-8, 1957

11. Stephens, F.D. Imperforate rectum. A New Surgical Technique, M.J. Australia 1:202-203, 1953

12. deVries, P.A., Peña, A.: Posterior Sagittal Anorectoplasty. J. Pediatr Surg 17(5):638-643, 1982

13. Peña, A., deVries, P.A.: Posterior Sagittal Anorectoplasty: Important Technical Considerations and New Application. J. Pediatr Surg 17(6):796-811, 1982

14. Hendren, W.H. Surgical Management of Urogenital Sinus Abnormalities. J. Pediatr Surg 12 (3) 339-357, 1977

15. Hendren, W.H. Urogenital Sinus and Anorectal Malformation: Experience with 22 cases. J. Pediatr Surg 15 (5) 628-641, 1980

16. Hendren, W.H. Further Experience in Reconstructive Surgery for Cloacal Anomalies. J Pediatr Surg 17 (6) 695-717, 1982

17. Thomas, Starzls. Ladd's Medal Recipient. Interview. Oral History Project. History Center. American Academy of Pediatrics 4, February 2007

18. Martinez, D. Juame, J., Stein, T., Peña, A.: The Effect of Costal Cartilage Resection on Chest Wall Development. Pediatr Surg Int 5:170-173, 1990

19. Nuss, D., Kelly, R. E. Jr., Croitoru, D. P., Katz, M. E. A 10-year review of a minimally invasive technique for the correction of pectus excavatum. J Pediatr Surg 33 (4) 545-552, 1998

20. Haight, C. and Towsley, H. A.: Congenital Atresia of the Esophagus with Tracheoesophageal Fistula. Extrapleural Ligation of Fistula and End to End Anastomosis of Esophageal Segments. Surg Gyn and Obst

LEGENDS OF FIGURES

1. Stephen's repair.
2. The new anatomic concept (left). The new repair (right).
3. Diagram of a cloaca (left). Diagram of a repaired cloaca (right).
4. Pectus excavatum. Before the operation.
5. Pectus excavatum. After the repair.
6. Long term results. Lack of growth of the chest.
7. Lateral films of the animal's chest comparing those with intact cartilages (left) with those with cartilages removed (right).
8. Same animals in anterior-posterior views.
9. The cartilage resection affected the growth of the entire chest as shown here. Specimen in a control animal (left). Animal that underwent a cartilage resection (right).

INDEX OF NAMES IN ALPHABETICAL ORDER

INDEX OF NAMES IN ORDER OF APPEARANCE